Reoperative Parathyroid Surgery

Ralph P. Tufano • Phillip K. Pellitteri
Editors

Reoperative Parathyroid Surgery

Techniques and Tips for Success

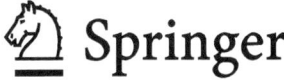 Springer

Editors
Ralph P. Tufano
Department of Otolaryngology – Head
and Neck Surgery
Johns Hopkins School of Medicine
Baltimore, MD, USA

Phillip K. Pellitteri
Department of Otolaryngology/Head
and Neck Surgery
Guthrie Health System
Sayre, PA, USA

ISBN 978-3-319-60722-1   ISBN 978-3-319-60723-8   (eBook)
DOI 10.1007/978-3-319-60723-8

Library of Congress Control Number: 2017951232

Printed on acid-free paper

This Springer imprint is published by Springer Nature
The registered company is Springer International Publishing AG
The registered company address is: Gewerbestrasse 11, 6330 Cham, Switzerland

Contents

Contributors

Nafi Aygun Radiology and Radiological Science-Neuroradiology, Department of Radiology, Johns Hopkins Medical Institutions, Baltimore, MD, USA

Jeffrey M. Bumpous Department of Otolaryngology, Head and Neck Surgery and Communicative Disorders, University of Louisville Hospital, Louisville, KY, USA

William R. Burns Department of Surgery, University of Michigan, Ann Arbor, MI, USA

Alan P.B. Dackiw Department of Surgery, University of Texas Southwestern Medical Center, Dallas, TX, USA

William S. Duke Department of Otolaryngology, Division of Endocrinology, Augusta University Thyroid and Parathyroid Center, Augusta University, Augusta, GA, USA

Salem I. Noureldine Division of Head and Neck Endocrine Surgery, Department of Otolaryngology – Head and Neck Surgery, Johns Hopkins Medical Institutions, Baltimore, MD, USA

Phillip K. Pellitteri Department of Otolaryngology/Head and Neck Surgery, Guthrie Health System, Sayre, PA, USA

Jonathon O. Russell Division of Head and Neck Endocrine Surgery, Department of Otolaryngology-Head and Neck Surgery, Johns Hopkins Medical Institutions, Baltimore, MD, USA

Michael C. Singer Division of Thyroid and Parathyroid Surgery, Department of Otolaryngology – Head and Neck Surgery, Henry Ford Health System, Detroit, MI, USA

David J. Terris Department of Otolaryngology, Division of Endocrinology, Augusta University Thyroid and Parathyroid Center, Augusta University, Augusta, GA, USA

Ralph P. Tufano Department of Otolaryngology – Head and Neck Surgery, Johns Hopkins School of Medicine, Baltimore, MD, USA

Mary Worthen Department of Otolaryngology, Head and Neck Surgery and Communicative Disorders, University of Louisville Hospital, Louisville, KY, USA

Chapter 1
Embryology and Anatomy of the Parathyroid Glands

William R. Burns and Alan P.B. Dackiw

Introduction

As with most surgical procedures, a surgeon's knowledge of the relevant anatomy is critical to the technical success of operations on the parathyroid glands. This knowledge must encompass more than just an understanding of the anatomy of the normal neck; it must also include an understanding of the variant anatomy and aberrant anatomic relationships that may be encountered. The process is reinforced by an appreciation and understanding of not only parathyroid anatomy but also parathyroid embryology. This chapter reviews the embryology and anatomy of the parathyroid glands in a clinically relevant manner. Furthermore, it details recent advances in our understanding of the molecular mechanisms of parathyroid development. Our aim is to reinforce the link between embryology and surgical anatomy in the context of parathyroid surgery such that parathyroid glands are successfully identified and operative morbidity is minimized. We also intend for this to serve as a reference and preface to the other chapters in this text.

W.R. Burns
Department of Surgery, University of Michigan,
1500 East Medical Center Drive, 3308 Cancer Center Floor, Ann Arbor, MI 48109, USA

A.P.B. Dackiw (✉)
Department of Surgery, University of Texas Southwestern Medical Center,
1801 Inwood Road, WA 3.416, Dallas, TX 75390, USA
e-mail: alan.dackiw@utsouthwestern.edu

© Springer International Publishing AG 2018   1
R.P. Tufano, P.K. Pellitteri (eds.), *Reoperative Parathyroid Surgery*,
DOI 10.1007/978-3-319-60723-8_1

A Historical Perspective

The importance of a detailed understanding of parathyroid embryology and anatomy is perhaps best appreciated by reviewing what may well be the most challenging case of persistent hyperparathyroidism in the surgical literature. Seventy-one years after Felix Mandl first removed a parathyroid tumor from his patient Albert J., a Viennese streetcar conductor with osteitis fibrosa cystica, the management of parathyroid disease remained a dilemma. So much so that at the 67th Annual Session of the Pacific Coast Surgical Association, Dr. Claude Organ noted:

> "William Halsted remarked once that 'It seems hardly creditable that the loss of bodies so tiny as the parathyroid should be followed by results so disastrous.' The second hardest decision is when to operate; the hardest decision is when to reoperate. It was inevitable with the dramatic increase in identification of the hypercalcemic syndromes and the increase in parathyroid surgery that we would eventually have to deal with the failed operation" [1].

While Mandl and his Austro-German colleagues were describing the physiology of hyperparathyroidism and anatomy of the parathyroid glands in the early twentieth century, parallel work was taking place across the Atlantic in the United States. Sea Captain Charles Martell, a World War I veteran, would become the first American patient diagnosed with hyperparathyroidism in 1926. Born in 1896 in Somerville, Massachusetts, Martell attended the Massachusetts Nautical School and graduated at the top of his class. He joined the World War I effort and was stationed near Liverpool. Following the armistice in 1918, he returned home to Massachusetts. At that time, he began experiencing back and groin pain that he attributed to his physical duties on the ship and rheumatism. The captain returned to the US Merchant Marines where he traveled throughout the world. At that time, his fellow officers noted that his physical appearance was beginning to change. He slowly lost height and his chest developed a pigeon deformity. Over time, he was no longer the athletic, vigorous, six-foot-one-inch man of the past. Meanwhile, he began passing what was described as "urinary gravel." Over the next several years, he was in and out of domestic and foreign hospitals due to multiple extremity fractures. In 1926, Captain Martell came under the care of Dr. Eugene F. DuBois at Bellevue Hospital in New York City. Unaware of Dr. Mandl's investigations of the patient Albert J., (who was found to have a parathyroid tumor associated with von Recklinghausen's disease as the cause of his osteitis fibrosa cystica) several years earlier in Austria, DuBois obtained a sample of blood from Martell. This revealed hypercalcemia. DuBois went on to identify that more calcium was being excreted than consumed by Martell. This was the first tentative diagnosis of hyperparathyroidism in the United States. Martell was referred to Massachusetts General Hospital in Boston where the senior thyroid surgeon, Edward P. Richardson, explored Martell's neck. A parathyroid gland was removed, but ultimately the pathology was normal and his hypercalcemia persisted. Over the next five neck explorations Martell underwent, his remaining parathyroid glands were removed without improvement in his disease. Finally, on November 2, 1932, at the seventh operation, Dr. Edward A. Churchill, Chief of Surgery at the Massachusetts General Hospital, performed an anterior mediastinotomy, which revealed a 2.5 cm parathyroid adenoma. Following this exploration and adenoma resection, Martell's serum calcium levels fell for the first time. Unfortunately, he developed hypocalcemia and tetany. Despite successful surgery, the years of chronic renal disease secondary to hypercalciuria and nephrocalcinosis caused his ultimate demise. Following a complicated postoperative course managing his fluids and electrolytes, he developed a left-sided kidney stone which became impacted and ultimately led to acute renal failure and subsequently his death. Despite the loss, Martell and his doctor's persistence in attempting to identify the underlying cause of his illness resulted in significant contributions to medical and surgical knowledge. In retrospect, over eight decades later, this ectopic parathyroid adenoma was in a seemingly likely location given our current knowledge of parathyroid embryology and anatomy. With this knowledge in mind and with the improved parathyroid imaging techniques we enjoy today, perhaps he would have been cured at his first operation [2, 3].

The unfortunate case of sea captain Charles Martell and his seven operations, before a mediastinal parathyroid adenoma was discovered, highlights the difficulty of treating this disease, as well as how current diagnostic modalities can help prevent nontherapeutic parathyroid surgery and the associated morbidity of such operations. As compared to over 80 years ago when Captain Martell presented with his ectopic parathyroid gland, improved knowledge of potential sites for ectopic and supernumerary glands along with superior imaging techniques provides surgeons the opportunity to avoid multiple unnecessary operations. In view of this, it cannot be overemphasized how critical knowledge of the embryologic development and anatomic distribution of the parathyroid glands is for the surgeon treating patients with recurrent or ectopic disease in striving to perform a low morbidity operation.

Embryology and Anatomy

Like the thyroid gland (an outpouching of pharyngeal endoderm), the epithelial origin of the parathyroids is also the pharyngeal endoderm. The parathyroid glands, however, develop from the third and fourth pharyngeal pouches beginning in the fifth week of gestation (Fig. 1.1). The inferior glands are derived from the dorsal tip of the third pharyngeal pouch, as is the thymus. This collection of tissue, often referred to as the "parathymus," descends anteroinferiorly until the parathyroids find their position at the lower border of the thyroid lobes; the thymus, however, continues inferiorly into the anterior mediastinum. The superior glands, on the other hand, arise from the fourth pharyngeal pouch. By the sixth week of gestation, these superior glands separate from their origin, migrate inferiorly, and come to rest just superior and medial to the inferior glands. Their usual location approximates the point at which the inferior thyroid artery enters the thyroid gland or at which the inferior thyroid artery crosses the recurrent laryngeal nerve. Therefore, while the inferior glands begin more superiorly, they pass the superior glands on their descent and are named "inferior" based on their mature location (Fig. 1.2).

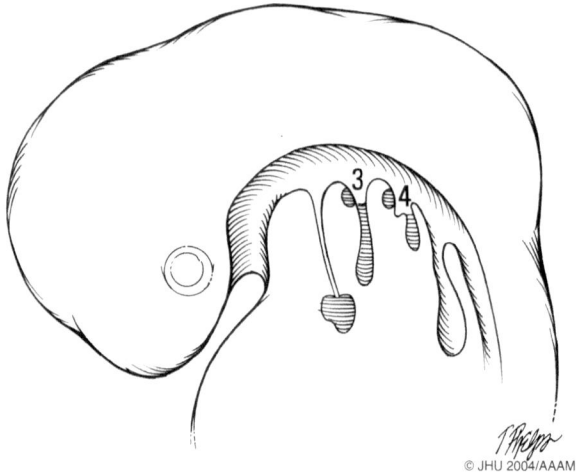

Fig. 1.1 Migration of the thyroid, parathyroids, and pharyngeal pouch derivatives. The thyroid, parathyroid glands, and ultimobranchial bodies migrate inferiorly from their origin in the embryo. Courtesy of Tim Phelps © JHU/AAAM 2004, Department of Art as Applied to Medicine, The Johns Hopkins University School of Medicine

To elaborate and consider this in further detail, the entire head and neck region is derived from ectoderm, mesoderm, endoderm, and neural crest-derived cells. During the fourth and fifth weeks of development, the pharyngeal, or branchial arches arise from a core of mesoderm that is lined internally by endoderm of the primitive foregut and externally by surface ectoderm. Bars of mesenchymal tissue become separated by deep grooves known as branchial clefts. Simultaneously, five pairs of outpockets develop along the lateral walls of the most cranial portion of the foregut, the pharyngeal gut. These outpockets are known as the pharyngeal pouches (Figs. 1.1 and 1.2). Unique to both the third and fourth pharyngeal pouches, dorsal and ventral wings develop bilaterally [4–7].

During the fifth week of embryogenesis, the endodermally derived epithelium of the third pouch differentiates. The dorsal wing becomes the right and left inferior parathyroid glands, respectively, while the ventral wing forms a portion of the thymus that will later coalesce. Bilaterally, the gland primordia lose their connection with the pharyngeal wall in order to allow migration in a caudal and medial direction. The rapid movement of the paired thymic counterparts toward the anterior mediastinum in the thorax draws the inferior parathyroid glands with them (Fig. 1.2). Upon arrival in the thorax, the thymic counterparts fuse to form the final gland. Occasionally, this fails to occur completely, and a tail of thymic remnant may persist in the thyroid gland (derived as noted from an outpouching of the pharyngeal endoderm; foramen cecum in the adult) or as an independent island of thymic tissue in the neck. As the thymus descends, the inferior parathyroid glands migrate to their final location most commonly along the inferoposterior aspect of the thyroid gland. However, the migration is highly variable and the glands can be found at any location

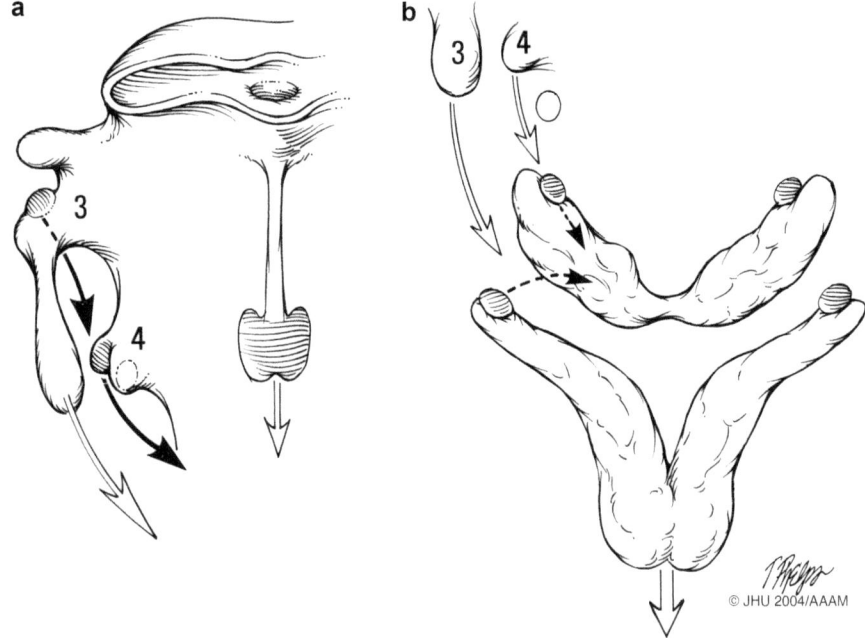

Fig. 1.2 (**a**) The upper (IV) and lower (III) parathyroids exchange position as they migrate; parathyroid III becomes the inferior parathyroid, whereas parathyroid IV becomes the superior parathyroid. (**b**) The inferior parathyroid has a more variable location due to its longer migration and may commonly be found in the thyrothymic ligament or the thymus itself. Courtesy of Tim Phelps © JHU/AAAM 2004, Department of Art as Applied to Medicine, The Johns Hopkins University School of Medicine

from intrathyroidally to along the thyrothymic ligament to within the thymus if the dorsal and ventral wings of the third pouch fail to separate. This variability of each parathyroid gland is independent of the migration of the contralateral gland, thereby resulting in significant variability in adults. Nonetheless, the lower parathyroid gland is typically located anterior to the recurrent laryngeal nerve.

Similar to the third pouch, the fourth pharyngeal pouch also divides into a dorsal and ventral wing. Again, the dorsal wing forms parathyroidal nests that give rise to the superior parathyroid glands bilaterally. The ventral wings develop into the ulti-mobranchial body, which will later become incorporated into the thyroid gland and become the parafollicular or C cells that secrete calcitonin. The superior parathyroid glands invaginate and attach themselves to the caudally migrating thyroid gland (Figs. 1.1 and 1.2). Ultimately, the bilateral superior parathyroid glands usually locate symmetrically, either in close association with the superior pole of the thyroid gland or occasionally within the thyroid gland itself. A majority of the superior glands are posterolateral in location and lie just above or just below the intersection of the inferior thyroid artery and the recurrent laryngeal nerve but posterior to the recurrent nerve.

It is the numerous variations in embryologic pharyngeal pouch development that result in the wide variability and the "predictable unpredictability" of parathyroid gland anatomy ranging from supernumerary glands and variable locations within the neck to intrathyroidal and, occasionally, ectopic sites such as those in the mediastinum. As a result of these substantial variations, the treatment of hyperparathyroidism may be complicated by recurrent or refractory disease.

Applied Anatomy and Embryology: Clinically Relevant Abnormalities

As a result of the embryologic development discussed above, parathyroid glands are often found in abnormal or ectopic locations or may be supernumerary (Fig. 1.3). The inferior parathyroids have the greatest irregularity in their position, based on their long path of descent. Ectopic inferior glands may be found in the lower pole of the thyroid lobes, or they may continue to descend with the thymus and continue into the mediastinal structures such as the thymus or thyrothymic ligament. Alternatively, the inferior parathyroid glands may fail to descend beyond the angle of the mandible or be along their proximal path of descent along or in the carotid sheath. Conversely, ectopic superior glands are usually within two centimeters of their expected location and usually found in a more dorsal position than the inferior

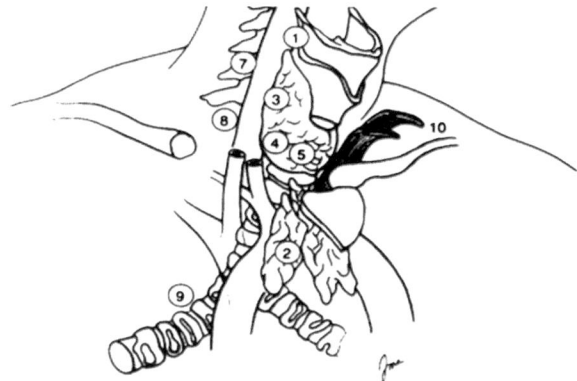

Fig. 1.3 Locations of normal, missed, and ectopic parathyroid glands. The single most common site of missed adenoma glands was in the tracheal esophageal groove in the posterior superior mediastinum (27%). The most common ectopic sites for parathyroid adenomas are thymus (17%), intrathyroidal (10%), undescended glands (8.6%), carotid sheath (3.6%), and the retroesophageal space (3.2%). Overall, the distribution of the 215 abnormal parathyroid adenomas resected in this series: (1) tracheoesophageal groove ($n = 59$; 27%); (2) anterior mediastinum/thymus ($n = 38$; 18%); (3) normal upper ($n = 28$; 13%); (4) normal lower ($n = 26$; 12%); (5) intrathyroid ($n = 22$; 10%); (6) undescended ($n = 18$; 8.4%); (7) carotid sheath ($n = 8$; 3.7%); (8) retroesophageal ($n = 7$; 3.3%); (9) other mediastinal ($n = 3$; 1.4%); (10) strap muscles ($n = 3$; 1.4%); (11) other ($n = 3$; 1.4%). Adapted from [8]

glands; the superior glands are often found in such positions as the retropharyngeal or retroesophageal spaces (Fig. 1.3). The single most common site of missed glands in a large series was in the tracheoesophageal groove in the posterior superior mediastinum (27%). The most common ectopic sites for parathyroid adenomas are also in the thymus (17%), intrathyroidal (10%), undescended glands (8.6%), carotid sheath (3.6%), and the retroesophageal space (3.2%) [8].

Supernumerary parathyroid glands may have an even wider variance in location. These glands are thought to develop from fragments of the pharyngeal pouches or primordial parathyroid tissue. These small clusters of cells migrate with surrounding structures and may develop in the lateral neck or lower mediastinum.

Molecular Biology of Parathyroid Development

The molecular mechanisms and biology of parathyroid development has been best described by the study of parathyroid developmental anomalies in humans. These anomalies, which result in hypoparathyroidism, may occur in up to one in 4000 live births and have been linked to defects in genes encoding putative transcription factors and/or enhancer proteins which impact parathyroid development. Several of the well-described syndromes are listed here, with the associated gene in parenthesis: DiGeorge syndrome (TBX1); hypothyroidism, deafness, and renal anomalies (HDR) syndrome (GATA3); isolated hypoparathyroidism (GCMB); X-linked recessive hypoparathyroidism (SOX3); and pluriglandular autoimmune hypoparathyroidism (AIRE1). These genes, as well as members of the homeobox (Hox) and paired box (Pax) families, have also been associated with parathyroid developmental abnormalities in mice [9]. This is not surprising, as the murine parathyroid glands have a similar embryologic development as human parathyroid glands. However, it should be noted that parathyroids in mice develop from only the endoderm of the third pharyngeal pouch and from neural crest cells arising from the embryonic mid- and hindbrain. As we have already reviewed, the parathyroids in humans develop from endoderm of the third and fourth pharyngeal pouches. In addition, recent studies have also demonstrated that fish express parathyroid hormone [10]. This is contrary to the long-held view that the earliest animals to possess parathyroid hormone were amphibians. In fact, two species of fish have been shown to express parathyroid hormone; however, the source and physiological function of this peptide in fish remains an area of ongoing investigation. As noted in the above murine and human studies, there is strong recent evidence that regulation and development of the parathyroid gland in mammals is controlled by a cascade of genes. A number of these regulatory factors that have been identified using genetically modified mouse models or as studying genes causing associated with human disease (including Gcm2/GCMB, Pax1/PAX1 and Pax9/PAX9, Hox3a/HOX3A, Tbx1/TBX1, Gata3/ATAGATA3, Tbce/TBCE, Sox3/SOX3, Eya1, and Six1/4) have also been found to be expressed in fish. While these parathyroid hormone expression genes are present in fish, their function remains unclear. Ongoing research promises to provide greater detail as to how this cascade of genes regulates parathyroid development.

Conclusion

In order that morbidity be reduced, and complications during parathyroid surgery (especially reoperative parathyroid surgery) be avoided in pursuit of achieving high rates of success in operations for hyperparathyroidism, the parathyroid surgeon must have an intimate understanding of the applied surgical embryology and anatomy of these endocrine glands. This current understanding of anatomy and embryology clearly would have benefitted Charles Martell, in helping to avoid most of his seven operations and his untimely death. Recent studies, as summarized above, have given us an even greater insight into the molecular factors important in parathyroid gland development and greater knowledge regarding gland migration, development, and morphogenesis. Ongoing and future work may provide even greater information regarding parathyroid anatomy and biology to further aid the parathyroid surgeon and patients afflicted with parathyroid disease.

References

1. Shen W, et al. Reoperation for persistent or recurrent primary hyperparathyroidism. Arch Surg. 1996;131(8):861–7. discussion 867–9
2. Albright F. A page out of the history of hyperparathyroidism. J Clin Endocrinol. 1948;8(8):637–57.
3. Bauer W, Federman DD. Hyperparathyroidism epitomized: the case of captain Charles E. Martell Metabol. 1962;11:21–9.
4. Sadler T. Langman's medical embryology. In: Head and neck. Baltimore, MD: Williams & Wilkins; 1995. p. 312–46.
5. Larsen WJ, Sherman LS, Potter SS, Scott WJ. Development of the head, the neck, the eyes, and the ears. In: Larsen WJ, Sherman LS, Potter SS, Scott WJ, editors. Human Embryology. 3rd ed. Philadelphia, PA: Churchill Livingstone; 2001.
6. Skandalakis JE, Gray SW, Todd NW. The pharynx and its derivatives. In: Skandalakis JE, Gray SW, editors. Embryology for surgeons: the embryological basis for the treatment of congenital anomalies. 2nd ed. Baltimore, MD: Williams and Wilkins; 1994. p. 17–64.
7. Mansberger AR, Wei JP. Surgical embryology and anatomy of the thyroid and parathyroid glands. Surgical clinics of North America, John E. Skandalakis. W.B. Saunders Company: Philadelphia, PA. 1993; 73: 4. pp 727-746.
8. Jaskowiak N, Norton JA, Alexander HR, Doppman JL, Shawker T, Skarulis M, Marx S, Spiegel A, Fraker DL. A prospective trial evaluating a standard approach to reoperation for missed parathyroid adenoma. Ann Surg. 1996;224(3):308–22.
9. Grigorieva IV, Thakker RV. Transcription factors in parathyroid development: lessons from hypoparathyroid disorders. Ann N Y Acad Sci. 2011;1237(1):24–38.
10. Zajac JD, Danks JA. The development of the parathyroid gland: from fish to human. Curr Opin Nephrol Hypertens. 2008;17(4):353–6.

Chapter 2
Maximizing the Success of Initial Parathyroid Surgery

William S. Duke and David J. Terris

Introduction

Parathyroid surgery has changed significantly over the past two decades. An operation that once required a large incision, exploration of all four glands, postoperative drainage, and inpatient management and was frequently associated with serious complications has largely been replaced by safe, minimally invasive, single-gland procedures that can be performed on an outpatient basis. This revolution has been facilitated by a number of factors. Improvements in the understanding of the complex relationships between parathyroid, renal, and bone physiology and routine annual evaluation of serum calcium levels have changed the classic presentation of hyperparathyroidism (HPT), allowing the disease to be diagnosed earlier and giving rise to a predominantly asymptomatic patient phenotype [1]. Advancements in preoperative imaging modalities make it possible to identify the single hyperfunctional gland in many cases, allowing targeted surgery with the assistance of adjuncts such as intraoperative ultrasound and endoscopic visualization [2]. Biochemical cure can be confirmed with intraoperative parathyroid hormone (IOPTH) assays, eliminating the need for four-gland exploration in most instances and reducing the risk of hypoparathyroidism [3].

Despite these advances, parathyroid surgery remains an endeavor fraught with potential pitfalls. The biochemical diagnosis may be uncertain or even incorrect in some patients. Preoperative imaging studies, required for targeted minimally invasive procedures, may be nonlocalizing, discordant, or misleading. Parathyroidectomy is unique in that locating the diseased organ(s) may be difficult, and grossly differentiating normal from abnormal tissue may challenge even the most experienced

W.S. Duke • D.J. Terris (✉)
Department of Otolaryngology, Division of Endocrinology, Augusta University Thyroid and Parathyroid Center, Augusta University, 1120 15th Street, BP-4109, Augusta, GA 30912, USA
e-mail: dterris@augusta.edu

© Springer International Publishing AG 2018
R.P. Tufano, P.K. Pellitteri (eds.), *Reoperative Parathyroid Surgery*,
DOI 10.1007/978-3-319-60723-8_2

surgeons. Once identified, the amount of abnormal parathyroid tissue to be excised or preserved is somewhat subjective yet has a profound impact on the surgical outcome. Determining when to terminate the operation is also dependent on the experience of the surgeon, as there is no absolute operative finding or IOPTH threshold that guarantees a cure. This chapter addresses these challenges and describes specific steps to maximize the success of initial parathyroid surgery, in the hopes of avoiding the need for reoperation.

Preoperative Factors

Diagnostic Dilemmas

Establishing the diagnosis of HPT is the most important preoperative step in successful parathyroid surgery. While the diagnosis is usually straightforward in patients with high serum calcium and parathyroid hormone (PTH) levels, there are times when the diagnosis is less clear. Hypercalcemia is generally first discovered on a routine chemistry panel. Often, this prompts later assessment of an isolated PTH level, which may be "normal." This scenario is misleading because while serum calcium levels change relatively slowly over hours or days, the half-life of the PTH molecule is much shorter, only 3–5 min [4, 5]. Additionally, small changes in the serum calcium values may lead to relatively larger changes in the PTH level [6]. Because of these factors, the serum calcium and PTH levels should be obtained simultaneously to provide a clear picture of their relationship.

There are three occasions in which the calcium/PTH relationship may be confounding. The first of these is the scenario in which the serum calcium is elevated but the PTH level is within the normal range, generally around 40–60 pg/mL [7]. The PTH should be suppressed to very low levels in patients with non-parathyroid-mediated hypercalcemia [8]. These patients, as well as patients with concurrent high-normal calcium and high-normal PTH levels [9], are said to have "inappropriately normal" PTH levels, indicating that at least one parathyroid gland is not completely suppressed by the elevated calcium level and is therefore autonomously functioning.

Another atypical phenotype, normocalcemic hyperparathyroidism, has also been described. This condition is characterized by consistent elevations in the PTH level despite normal serum and ionized calcium levels after other causes of secondary HPT have been excluded [10]. Though this condition and its potential morbidity are still incompletely understood, approximately one quarter of patients with this condition may progress to overt hypercalcemic HPT [11]. Long-term observation is warranted in many of these patients, although surgery may be offered in selected patients, particularly if they develop symptoms of classical hyperparathyroidism or have positive imaging findings [10–12].

Familial hypocalciuric hypercalcemia (FHH) may also present a diagnostic dilemma. This rare autosomal dominant disorder is due to abnormalities in the calcium-sensing receptor (*CASR*) gene. The resultant abnormal calcium-sensing receptors expressed on parathyroid and renal cells have reduced sensitivity to calcium levels, resulting in mild hypercalcemia with normal to slightly elevated PTH levels and normal phosphate levels [13]. Preoperative screening with a 24 h urinary calcium measurement to determine the calcium/creatinine clearance ratio (CCCR) helps differentiate most patients with primary HPT (PHPT) from those with FHH. The urinary calcium level is normal to elevated in patients with PHPT, while it is low to low normal in those with FHH. The urine volume should be over 1000 mL for a 24 h period for the specimen to be considered adequate for interpretation. Additionally, the CCCR is greater than 0.02 in patients with PHPT and typically less than 0.01 in FHH. The diagnosis becomes less clear when the CCCR is between 0.01 and 0.02, so patients with a CCCR in this range may benefit from *CASR* mutational analysis to clearly establish the diagnosis [14, 15]. Securing the diagnosis is critical, as patients with FHH will not benefit from surgical intervention [16].

In addition to assessing serum calcium and PTH levels, other laboratory values may be of importance in securing the diagnosis, evaluating for confounding factors, and assessing for the presence of secondary hyperparathyroidism. An ionized calcium should be obtained. Both the ionized calcium and serum calcium are usually elevated in PHPT, but in some cases of PHPT, the ionized calcium will be elevated even though the serum calcium is normal [17]. Renal function (creatinine and glomerular filtration rate) and 25-OH vitamin D should be measured to evaluate for causes of secondary HPT. An albumin level helps determine the reliability of the serum calcium measurement and permits calculation of a corrected calcium level if the albumin is abnormal. Alkaline phosphatase is a useful marker of bone turnover, and assessment of serum phosphorous is valuable in patients with renal hyperparathyroidism or when the diagnosis of PHPT is unclear. Finally, temporarily halting medications associated with PTH elevations, such as lithium, bisphosphonates, and thiazide diuretics, may assist in securing the diagnosis [10].

Surgical Candidacy

Once the diagnosis of PHPT is confirmed, a decision must be made as to whether or not the patient needs an operation. Patients with symptomatic PHPT [18], severe renal hyperparathyroidism [19], and persistent tertiary hyperparathyroidism [20] should be referred for surgery if there are no contradictory medical comorbidities. Guidelines exist to help manage the majority of patients with PHPT who now present with "asymptomatic" disease [18, 21]. Some of these patients may be candidates for observation or medical therapy, but regardless of their symptoms (or lack thereof), every patient diagnosed with PHPT should be offered the option of surgical consultation, since surgery presents the only opportunity to cure the disease [21].

Preoperative Localization

Preoperative localization is a fundamental component of minimally invasive focused parathyroid surgery, but these studies must be applied appropriately and interpreted thoughtfully to maximize their clinical utility. The diagnosis of PHPT is biochemical, not radiologic, and the purpose of preoperative localization is only to plan and guide the operation [21]. Therefore, preoperative localization studies should only be obtained after confirming the diagnosis with laboratory testing and after deciding to proceed with surgery. Conversely, it is the patient and their disease that determine surgical candidacy, and surgical consultation should not be withheld if localization studies are negative.

Localization studies are most often performed with imaging modalities such as technetium-99 m (^{99m}Tc)-sestamibi (sestamibi) [22] and high-resolution ultrasound (US) [23]. More recently, four-dimensional computed tomography (CT) scanning has been employed, especially where sestamibi scanning has yielded suboptimal results [24, 25]. The quality of preoperative imaging, particularly sestamibi, is volume and technique dependent, with busy centers producing the most reliable results [26]. However, surgeons are encouraged to personally review all imaging findings and be aware of potential imaging pitfalls. We will discuss the two most common imaging studies obtained when considering focused surgery for primary hyperparathyroidism.

Sestamibi

^{99m}Tc-sestamibi is a radiopharmaceutical agent that is preferentially taken up by cells with high mitochondrial activity, such as the thyroid and parathyroid glands [27]. It is retained longer by hyperfunctional parathyroid tissue than by the thyroid, and therefore a dual-phase study after a washout period may reveal a parathyroid adenoma. The timing of the second study acquisition is important, with optimal results obtained after a 2 h period [28]. Images obtained after this time interval risk missing the lesion [29], so surgeons should pay close attention to when the second phase of the scan was performed if the study is negative. Occasionally the sestamibi will rapidly wash out of a parathyroid adenoma, resulting in a negative scan even at 2 h [30]. In either of these situations, careful scrutiny of the early-phase image may reveal subtle asymmetry in the height of the thyroid lobes, which may point toward the location of an adenoma (Fig. 2.1) [31].

Another pitfall in sestamibi interpretation involves determining the vertical location of a hyperfunctioning gland and distinguishing an inferior adenoma from a superior one that has descended low in the neck. These overly descended superior adenomas may be mistaken for inferior gland adenomas on two-dimensional planar imaging (Fig. 2.2) [32]. Surgeons may miss these adenomas, which are always posterior to the coronal plane of the recurrent laryngeal nerve, if the dissection is not continued deep enough in a paraesophageal or retroesophageal plane. Additionally, surgeons acting on misleading information from the planar imaging may remove the

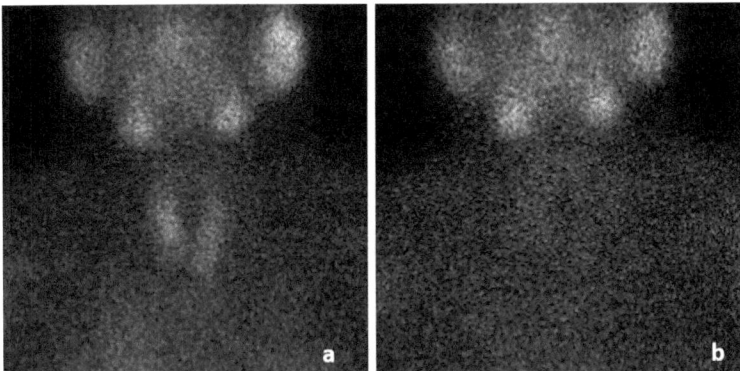

Fig. 2.1 Early (**a**) and late (**b**) planar two-dimensional ^{99m}Tc-sestamibi scan showing complete washout on the late-phase image. Careful evaluation of the early-phase image shows asymmetric inferior extension of the left thyroid, suggesting the presence of a left inferior parathyroid adenoma, which was confirmed at surgery

normal inferior gland. If the inferior gland appears normal, it should be preserved, and the surgeon should dissect deeper into the neck to identify the overly descended superior adenoma. This condition may be more readily predicted by adding single photon emission computed tomography (SPECT) coupled with computed tomography (CT) to the preoperative imaging regimen, which gives more precise anatomic localization of these deep adenomas (Fig. 2.3) [33].

Ultrasound

Ultrasound, which is also frequently employed to localize anatomically abnormal parathyroid glands, offers a number of advantages, particularly when performed by the operating surgeon [34]. It is quick and noninvasive, avoids radiation, and permits differentiation between thyroid nodules, lymph nodes, and parathyroid lesions (Fig. 2.4) [2, 35]. Surgeon-performed ultrasound in the operating room immediately before incision allows the surgeon to triangulate the location of the adenoma relative to the surrounding structures, facilitating the subsequent dissection. Though the overall sensitivity of ultrasound for detecting parathyroid lesions is only 76% [36], experienced parathyroid surgeons know that there is often information to be gleaned in even "negative" studies.

Ultrasound reports, especially when they reportedly fail to definitively identify a parathyroid adenoma, deserve careful scrutiny to ensure that a parathyroid lesion is not mistaken for a "posterior" hypoechoic thyroid nodule. There will often be a rim of normal thyroid tissue along the deep surface of a posterior thyroid nodule, which will be absent when the hypoechoic lesion "just posterior to the thyroid capsule" is in fact the parathyroid adenoma. Biopsy of these posterior thyroid "nodules" may be reported as "suspicious for follicular neoplasm." Even in this context, the lesion may still represent a parathyroid adenoma, which is difficult to distinguish from

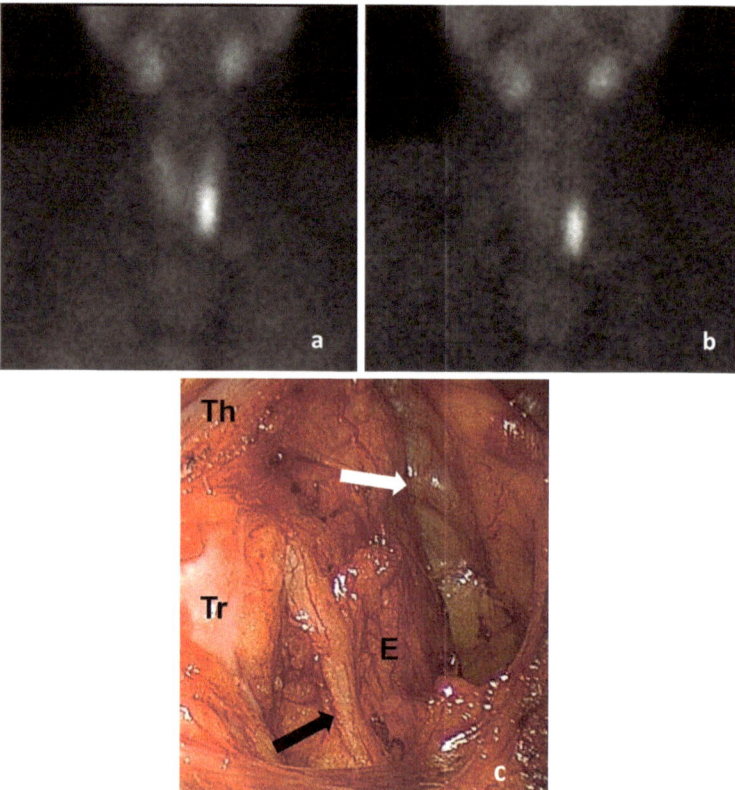

Fig. 2.2 Early (**a**) and late (**b**) planar two-dimensional ^{99m}Tc-sestamibi scan showing a suspected left inferior parathyroid adenoma. (**c**) An ectopic, overly descended superior parathyroid adenoma (*white arrow*) was identified at surgery, deep to the recurrent laryngeal nerve (*black arrow*) and esophagus (E). *Th* thyroid, *Tr* trachea

Fig. 2.3 Single photon emission computed tomography/computed tomography (SPECT/CT) image showing a retrotracheal parathyroid adenoma (*arrow*)

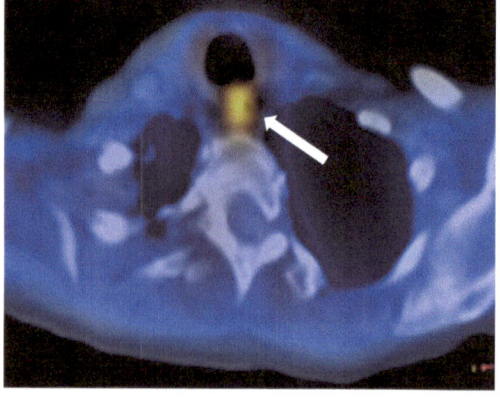

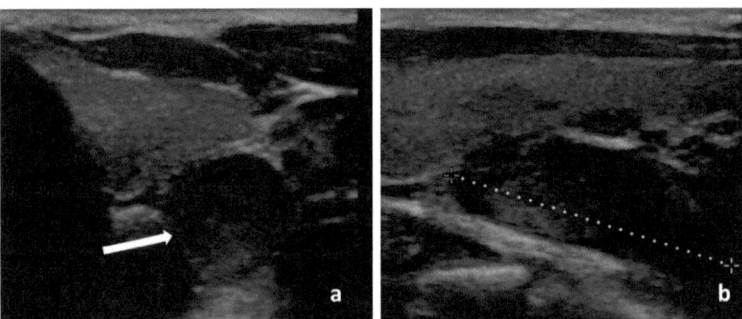

Fig. 2.4 Transverse (**a**) and longitudinal (**b**) ultrasound images showing a left inferior parathyroid adenoma. Parathyroid adenomas are generally rounded or ovoid on transverse view (**a**, *arrow*) and ovoid with a polar vascular supply on longitudinal imaging (**b**, *dotted line*). This distinguishes them from lymph nodes, which are more rounded and have a central hilar vascular supply

thyroid tissue on cytopathology [37]. If there is suspicion that a "thyroid" nodule might actually be a parathyroid adenoma, then a washout of the aspirate may be sent for PTH analysis. While this is rarely necessary and generally reserved for reoperative cases, aspiration of parathyroid tissue usually reveals an unequivocally high PTH level in the thousands, while aspiration of thyroid or lymph node tissue typically results in levels below 100 pg/mL [38]. Truly negative ultrasound studies also may offer helpful information and hint to the surgeon that the adenoma may be small, deep, or ectopic, or that multigland disease may be present [39, 40].

Intraoperative Factors

Preoperative Ultrasound

Performing an ultrasound examination just prior to the start of the operation can be of tremendous value in pinpointing the location of a parathyroid adenoma. Cervical landmarks and tissue relationships change considerably between the upright, supine, and final surgical position [41], and muscle relaxation from the anesthetic may improve the image quality. This examination confirms the location of the adenoma and its relationship to the surrounding structures, which allows focused dissection to the adenoma.

Parathyroid Identification

Successful parathyroid surgery requires a complete command of parathyroid embryology and cervical anatomy, which has been covered in Chap. 1. Parathyroid tissue may be present in ectopic locations in up to 20% of patients [42, 43], and surgeons must be prepared to explore these sites if a parathyroid gland is not found in its expected position. Ectopic superior glands may be found in paraesophageal, retro-esophageal, retropharyngeal, or retrolaryngeal sites or within the carotid sheath or posterior mediastinum [43–45]. They may be overly descended in a deep location or undescended near the hyoid [32]. Ectopic inferior glands are most frequently located in the thymus, thyrothymic ligament, or anterior mediastinum, though they can exist anywhere between the skull base and anterior mediastinum, including the pyriform sinus, submandibular region, and aorticopulmonary window or pericardium [43, 44, 46–48]. Both superior or inferior parathyroid glands may be found within the thyroid parenchyma [45]. Ultrasound may be beneficial in identifying intrathyroidal adenomas [48]. Bilateral venous sampling of the internal jugular veins for IOPTH assessment may help identify which side of the neck harbors the hyperfunctional gland if abnormal parathyroid tissue is not readily identifiable [49]. A difference in the PTH level of more than 5% between the two aspirates has been shown to predict the side of the hyperfunctional tissue [50].

Surgeons must also be able to distinguish parathyroid tissue from surrounding fatty, lymphatic, thymic, and thyroid tissue and be able to discern normal parathyroid glands from abnormal ones. Normal parathyroid glands are typically flat, 3–8 mm long, with an average weight of 40 mg and a light brown to tobacco color [44, 51]. They are usually surrounded by or capped with fat. Parathyroid adenomas and hyperplastic glands are typically larger, more rounded or nodular, and rubbery and have a darker red-brown color. Bloodless dissection is essential in parathyroid surgery, as any bleeding will stain the tissue and make it challenging to differentiate the parathyroid glands from the surrounding tissue.

Confirming Surgical Cure

Bilateral neck exploration (BNE) with visual confirmation of all four parathyroid glands has been the gold standard for parathyroid surgery for nearly 100 years [52, 53]. This procedure, which requires surgeons to compare the appearance of the glands and determine which one(s) to resect based on their gross appearance, has a long-term cure rate greater than 95% in experienced hands [54]. More recently, unilateral and minimally invasive single-gland procedures have been developed that share the same cure rates as BNE [18, 55]. However, since visual assessment of all parathyroid glands is not performed in these more focused approaches, the use of intraoperative adjuncts such as IOPTH monitoring or radioguided surgery using a handheld gamma probe is recommended to ensure complete removal of all hyperfunctional parathyroid tissue [56, 57]. Though radioguided parathyroid surgery has been successfully routinely implemented in some practices [57], other groups have found it cumbersome and unhelpful in many cases and reserve its use for selected reoperative procedures [58]. It is reported to be associated with a 6% long-term recurrence rate, calling into question its value in parathyroid surgery [59].

IOPTH assessment is the most common method of assessing biochemical cure in minimally invasive parathyroid surgery, and multiple algorithms for predicting successful surgery have been proposed [56, 60]. Although the Miami criterion, which predicts postoperative normocalcemia when the IOPTH value decreases ≥50% from the highest of either the pre-incisional or the pre-excision level 10 min after removal of all the hyperfunctional parathyroid tissue [60], is often reported in the literature, many surgeons have adopted a stricter threshold that requires the PTH level to also drop into the normal or low-normal range prior to terminating the operation in patients with PHPT [56, 61]. Additionally, obtaining IOTPH values 5, 10, and sometimes 15 min after adenoma excision allows the degradation trajectory to be trended to ensure that there is no additional hyperfunctional tissue [2].

Failed Exploration

Parathyroidectomy may be both one of the most rewarding and most challenging surgical endeavors. Despite a high success rate with either four-gland or focused techniques, operative failures persist. If all four parathyroid glands cannot be identified with BNE or if IOTPH levels fail to decline as expected, it is important for surgeons to first verify their findings and "know what they know." If the surgeon has any doubts, suspected parathyroid tissue may sampled away from its polar blood supply to be sent for frozen section confirmation that it is indeed parathyroid tissue and not lymph node, fat, thyroid, or thymus. While frozen section analysis can generally distinguish between parathyroid and non-parathyroid tissue, it is not able to reliably and consistently differentiate a normocellular parathyroid gland from one that is adenomatous or hyperplastic [62, 63]. Aspiration of the excised tissue for IOPTH analysis is also beneficial in confirming the presence of parathyroid tissue and can be performed more quickly than frozen section analysis [63]. Once the identity of the excised tissue is confirmed, a diligent search for the missing, and presumably hyperfunctional, tissue can commence. The preoperative localization studies should be reviewed, and the early- and late-phase sestamibi images, if available in the operating room, should be carefully scrutinized for any hint of additional abnormal foci. Attention should first be turned to the side of the neck where both glands have not yet been found. If more than one gland has not been identified or if IOPTH levels remain elevated after finding all four glands, simultaneous bilateral venous sampling of the internal jugular vein may help guide the dissection.

Each side of the neck should be carefully and fully explored. Identifying the recurrent laryngeal nerve will help guide the depth of dissection for a missing superior or inferior gland. If the inferior glands are missing, the thyrothymic tract and thymus should be explored or excised first. If the superior glands are missing, dissection should initially be directed deeply toward the esophagus or paraspinal musculature. If the missing glands are not found in these typical locations, all sites of potential ectopic tissue in the neck and upper mediastinum should be systematically evaluated. Intrathyroidal parathyroid adenomas have been reported in up to 7%

of cases [64]. Thyroidectomy is discouraged unless there is clear ultrasonographic evidence of a suspicious lesion within the thyroid and thorough exploration for the missing gland has failed. Consent for thyroidectomy should be obtained. If all four glands have been positively identified and the patient remains biochemically hyperparathyroid, then the possibility of supernumerary parathyroid glands should be considered [45]. If no further parathyroid tissue is identified or if the single hyperfunctional gland cannot be located, then the surgeon should consider intraoperative consultation with another experienced surgeon. Surgeons should refrain from removing any grossly or histologically normal parathyroid tissue. This "debulking" provides no benefit to the patient, as these glands are biochemically quiescent, and such an approach predisposes the patient to a risk of permanent hypoparathyroidism if an abnormal gland is removed during a subsequent operation.

If all of these efforts still fail to identify the source of the hyperparathyroidism, then the operation should be terminated, before any undue morbidity occurs. All confirmed normal parathyroid tissue should be marked with a clip or permanent suture away from its blood supply. The surgical findings should be fully documented in the operative report, including which glands were positively identified, which were missing, what was removed, and which areas were explored. Prior to parathyroid surgery, every patient should be counseled about the possibility of a negative exploration and the possible need for additional procedures. This counseling helps temper the patient's expectations of what may be perceived as "routine" or "minor" surgery and may help mitigate their disappointment if surgery is unsuccessful.

Conclusion

Although most patients with primary hyperparathyroidism can anticipate being cured after a single procedure, the sometimes challenging nature of parathyroid disease ensures that operative failures cannot be obviated completely. Surgeons should understand the potential causes of failed parathyroid surgery and be aware of possible pitfalls in the diagnosis and management of surgical parathyroid disease. Armed with a thorough understanding of parathyroid pathology, and with careful preoperative assessment, meticulous operative planning and execution, and thoughtful integration of surgical adjuncts, surgeons are well positioned to maximize the likelihood of successful initial parathyroid surgery.

References

1. Khan AA, Bilezikian JP, Potts JT Jr. The diagnosis and management of asymptomatic primary hyperparathyroidism revisited. J Clin Endocrinol Metab. 2009;94(2):333–4.
2. Terris DJ, Stack BC Jr, Gourin CG. Contemporary parathyroidectomy: exploiting technology. Am J Otolaryngol. 2007;28(6):408–14.

3. Karakas E, Schneider R, Rothmund M, Bartsch DK, Schlosser K. Initial surgery for benign primary hyperparathyroidism: an analysis of 1,300 patients in a teaching hospital. World J Surg. 2014;38(8):2011–8.
4. Bieglmayer C, Prager G, Niederle B. Kinetic analyses of parathyroid hormone clearance as measured by three rapid immunoassays during parathyroidectomy. Clin Chem. 2002;48(10):1731–8.
5. Leiker AJ, Yen TW, Eastwood DC, et al. Factors that influence parathyroid hormone half-life: determining if new intraoperative criteria are needed. JAMA Surg. 2013;148(7):602–6.
6. Felsenfeld AJ, Rodríguez M, Aguilera-Tejero E. Dynamics of parathyroid hormone secretion in health and secondary hyperparathyroidism. Clin J Am Soc Nephrol. 2007;2(6):1283–305.
7. Wallace LB, Parikh RT, Ross LV, et al. The phenotype of primary hyperparathyroidism with normal parathyroid hormone levels: how low can parathyroid hormone go? Surgery. 2011;150(6):1102–12.
8. Mirrakhimov AE. Hypercalcemia of malignancy: an update on pathogenesis and management. N Am J Med Sci. 2015;7(11):483–93.
9. Glendenning P, Gutteridge DH, Retallack RW, et al. High prevalence of normal total calcium and intact PTH in 60 patients with proven primary hyperparathyroidism: a challenge to current diagnostic criteria. Aust NZ J Med. 1998;28(2):173–8.
10. Eastell R, Brandi ML, Costa AG, et al. Diagnosis of asymptomatic primary hyperparathyroidism: proceedings of the fourth international workshop. J Clin Endocrinol Metab. 2014;99(10):3570–9.
11. Carneiro-Pla D, Solorzano C. A summary of the new phenomenon of normocalcemic hyperparathyroidism and appropriate management. Curr Opin Oncol. 2012;24(1):42–5.
12. Shindo M, Lee JA, Lubitz CC, et al. The changing landscape of primary, secondary, and tertiary hyperparathyroidism: highlights from the American College of Surgeons panel, "What's new for the surgeon caring for patients with hyperparathyroidism". J Am Coll Surg. 2016;222(6):1240–50.
13. Iacobone M, Carnaille B, Palazzo FF, Vriens M. Hereditary hyperparathyroidism-a consensus report of the European society of endocrine surgeons (ESES). Langenbeck's Arch Surg. 2015;400(8):867–86.
14. Bilezikian J, Potts J, Fuleihan G-H, et al. Summary statement from a workshop on asymptomatic primary hyperparathyroidism: a perspective for the 21st century. J Clin Endocrinol Metab. 2002;87(12):5353–61.
15. Christensen S, Nissen P, Vestergaard P, et al. Discriminative power of three indices of renal calcium excretion for the distinction between familial hypocalciuric hypercalcemia and primary hyperparathyroidism: a follow-up study on methods. Clin Endocrinol. 2008;69:713–20.
16. Varghese J, Rich T, Jimenez C. Benign familial hypocalciuric hypercalcemia. Endocr Pract. 2011;17(Suppl 1):13–7.
17. Wade TJ, Yen TW, Amin AL, Wang TS. Surgical management of normocalcemic primary hyperparathyroidism. World J Surg. 2012;36(4):761–6.
18. Udelsman R, Åkerström G, Biagini C, et al. The surgical management of asymptomatic primary hyperparathyroidism: proceedings of the fourth international workshop. J Clin Endocrinol Metab. 2014;99(10):3595–606.
19. Bratucu MN, Garofil ND, Radu PA, et al. Measurement of quality of life after total parathyroidectomy in patients with secondary hyperparathyroidism and end stage renal disease. Chirurgia (Bucur). 2015;110(6):511–7.
20. Cruzado JM, Moreno P, Torregrosa JV, et al. A randomized study comparing parathyroidectomy with cinacalcet for treating hypercalcemia in kidney allograft recipients with hyperparathyroidism. J Am Soc Nephrol. 2016;27(8):2487–9.
21. Bilezikian JP, Brandi ML, Eastell R, et al. Guidelines for the management of asymptomatic primary hyperparathyroidism: summary statement from the fourth international workshop. J Clin Endocrinol Metab. 2014;99(10):3561–9.

22. Taillefer R, Boucher Y, Potvin C, Lambert R. Detection and localization of parathyroid adenomas in patients with hyperparathyroidism using a single radionuclide imaging procedure with technetium-99m-sestamibi (double-phase study). J Nucl Med. 1992;33(10):1801–7.
23. Schenk WG III, Hanks JB, Smith PW. Surgeon-performed ultrasound for primary hyperparathyroidism. Am Surg. 2013;79(7):681–5.
24. Chazen JL, Gupta A, Dunning A, Phillips CD. Diagnostic accuracy of 4D-CT for parathyroid adenomas and hyperplasia. Am J Neuroradiol. 2012;33:429–33.
25. Hinson AM, Lee DR, Hobbs BA, et al. Preoperative 4D CT localization of nonlocalizing parathyroid adenomas by ultrasound and SPECT-CT. Otolaryngol Head Neck Surg. 2015;153(5):775–8.
26. Singer MC, Pucar D, Mathew M, Terris DJ. Improved localization of sestamibi imaging at high-volume centers. Laryngoscope. 2013;123(1):298–301.
27. Hetrakul N, Civelek AC, Stagg CA, Udelsman R. In vitro accumulation of technetium-99m-sestamibi in human parathyroid mitochondria. Surgery. 2001;130(6):1011–8.
28. Keane DF, Roberts G, Smith R, et al. Planar parathyroid localization scintigraphy: a comparison of subtraction and 1-, 2- and 3-h washout protocols. Nucl Med Commun. 2013;34(6):582–9.
29. Jofré J, González P, Massardo T, Zavala A. Optimal imaging time for delayed images in the diagnosis of abnormal parathyroid tissue with Tc-99m sestamibi. Clin Nucl Med. 1999;24(8):594–6.
30. Krausz Y, Shiloni E, Bocher M, et al. Diagnostic dilemmas in parathyroid scintigraphy. Clin Nucl Med. 2001;26(12):997–1001.
31. Nagar S, Walker DD, Embia O, et al. A novel technique to improve the diagnostic yield of negative sestamibi scans. Surgery. 2014;156(3):584–90.
32. Duke WS, Vernon HM, Terris DJ. Reoperative parathyroidectomy: overly descended superior adenoma. Otolaryngol Head Neck Surg. 2016;154(2):268–71.
33. Wong KK, Fig LM, Gross MD, Dwamena BA. Parathyroid adenoma localization with 99m Tc-sestamibi SPECT/CT: a meta-analysis. Nucl Med Commun. 2015;36(4):363–75.
34. Untch BR, Adam MA, Scheri RP, et al. Surgeon-performed ultrasound is superior to 99Tc-sestamibi scanning to localize parathyroid adenomas in patients with primary hyperparathyroidism: results in 516 patients over 10 years. J Am Coll Surg. 2011;212(4):522–9.
35. Kamaya A, Quon A, Jeffrey R. Sonography of the abnormal parathyroid gland. Ultrasound Q. 2006;22(4):253–62.
36. Cheung K, Wang T, Farrokhyar F, et al. A meta-analysis of preoperative localization techniques for patients with primary hyperparathyroidism. Ann Surg Oncol. 2012;19:577–83.
37. Odronic SI, Reynolds JP, Chute DJ. Cytologic features of parathyroid fine-needle aspiration on ThinPrep preparations. Cancer Cytopathol. 2014;122(9):678–84.
38. Bancos I, Grant CS, Nadeem S, et al. Risks and benefits of parathyroid fine-needle aspiration with parathyroid hormone washout. Endocr Pract. 2012;18(4):441–9.
39. Berber E, Parikh RT, Ballem N, et al. Factors contributing to negative parathyroid localization: an analysis of 1000 patients. Surgery. 2008;144(1):74–9.
40. Chandramohan A, Sathyakumar K, Irodi A, Abraham D, Paul MJ. Causes of discordant or negative ultrasound of parathyroid glands in treatment naïve patients with primary hyperparathyroidism. Eur J Radiol. 2012;81(12):3956–64.
41. Duke WS, Bush CM, Singer MC, et al. Incision planning in thyroid compartment surgery: getting it perfect. Endocr Pract. 2015;21(2):107–14.
42. Albuja-Cruz MB, Allan BJ, Parikh PP, Lew JI. Efficacy of localization studies and intraoperative parathormone monitoring in the surgical management of hyperfunctioning ectopic parathyroid glands. Surgery. 2013;154(3):453–60.
43. Phitayakorn R, McHenry CR. Incidence and location of ectopic abnormal parathyroid glands. Am J Surg. 2006;191(3):418–23.
44. Fancy T, Gallagher D, Hornig J. Surgical anatomy of the thyroid and parathyroid glands. Otolaryngol Clin N Am. 2010;43:221–7.
45. Mohebati A, Shaha AR. Anatomy of the thyroid and parathyroid glands and neurovascular relations. Clin Anat. 2012;25:19–31.

46. Wang C. The anatomic basis of parathyroid surgery. Ann Surg. 1976;183(3):271–5.
47. Gough I. Reoperative parathyroid surgery: the importance of ectopic location and multigland disease. ANZ J Surg. 2006;76(12):1048–50.
48. Roy M, Mazeh H, Chen H, Sippel RS. Incidence and localization of ectopic parathyroid adenomas in previously unexplored patients. World J Surg. 2013;37(1):102–6.
49. Franz RC, Ungerer JP, du Toit SA. Selective intra-operative internal jugular venous sampling for rapid immunoradiometric assay of intact parathyroid hormone during parathyroid surgery. S Afr Med J. 1997;87(9):1156.
50. Ito F, Sippel R, Lederman J, Chen H. The utility of intraoperative bilateral internal jugular venous sampling with rapid parathyroid hormone testing. Ann Surg. 2007;245(6):959–63.
51. Ritter H, Milas M. Bilateral parathyroid exploration for hyperparathyroidism. Oper Tech Otolaryngol. 2009;20:44–53.
52. Lorenz K, Nguyen-Thanh P, Dralle H. Unilateral open and minimally invasive procedures for primary hyperparathyroidism: a review of selective approaches. Langenbeck's Arch Surg. 2000;385(2):106–17.
53. Barczyński M, Gołkowski F, Nawrot I. The current status of intraoperative iPTH assay in surgery for primary hyperparathyroidism. Gland Surg. 2015;4(1):36–43.
54. Lee JA, Inabnet WB III. The surgeon's armamentarium to the surgical treatment of primary hyperparathyroidism. J Surg Oncol. 2005;89(3):130–5.
55. Westerdahl J, Bergenfelz A. Unilateral versus bilateral neck exploration for primary hyperparathyroidism: five-year follow-up of a randomized controlled trial. Ann Surg. 2007;246(6):976–80.
56. Barczynski M, Konturek A, Hubalewska-Dydejczyk A, Cichon S, Nowak W. Evaluation of Halle, Miami, Rome, and Vienna intraoperative iPTH assay criteria in guiding minimally invasive parathyroidectomy. Langenbeck's Arch Surg. 2009;394(5):843–9.
57. Adil E, Adil T, Fedok F, Kauffman G, Goldenberg D. Minimally invasive radioguided parathyroidectomy performed for primary hyperparathyroidism. Otolaryngol Head Neck Surg. 2009;141(1):34–8.
58. Noureldine SI, Gooi Z, Tufano RP. Minimally invasive parathyroid surgery. Gland Surg. 2015;4(5):410–9.
59. Norman J, Lopez J, Politz D. Abandoning unilateral parathyroidectomy: why we reversed our position after 15,000 parathyroid operations. J Am Coll Surg. 2012;214(3):260–9.
60. Carneiro DM, Solorzano CC, Nader MC, Ramirez M, Irvin GL III. Comparison of intraoperative iPTH assay (QPTH) criteria in guiding parathyroidectomy: which criterion is the most accurate? Surgery. 2003;134(6):973–9.
61. Lombardi CP, Raffaelli M, Traini E, et al. Intraoperative PTH monitoring during parathyroidectomy: the need for stricter criteria to detect multiglandular disease. Langenbeck's Arch Surg. 2008;393(5).639–45.
62. Johnson SJ. Changing clinicopathological practice in parathyroid disease. Histopathology. 2010;56(7):835–51.
63. Farrag T, Weinberger P, Seybt M, Terris DJ. Point-of-care rapid intraoperative parathyroid hormone assay of needle aspirates from parathyroid tissue: a substitute for frozen sections. Am J Otolaryngol. 2011;32(6):574–7.
64. Mazeh H, Kouniavsky G, Schneider DF, et al. Intrathyroidal parathyroid glands: small, but mighty (a Napoleon phenomenon). Surgery. 2012;152(6):1193–200.

Chapter 3
Indications for Reoperative Parathyroidectomy

Michael C. Singer

Some of the challenges of parathyroid surgery have been evident from the time of the first attempted parathyroidectomy in the early twentieth century. A number of these early patients with primary hyperparathyroidism experienced some form of surgical failure. In 1925, Albert Gahne underwent the first successful (initially at least) parathyroidectomy performed by Felix Mandl. Mr. Gahne responded well to the surgery; however, several years later, his hypercalcemia recurred, and he died shortly after a second attempted operation. Evidence suggests that his recurrent disease was a result of incomplete excision of the pathologic gland during his initial surgery [1]. In that same year, Oskar Hirsh was unable to find and remove the gland causing hypercalcemia in another patient. Several years later, Captain Charles Martell underwent the first of six failed parathyroid operations, before a mediastinal adenoma was eventually identified and removed in a seventh attempt.

These problems of persistent and recurrent disease continue to be the burden of all surgeons performing parathyroid surgery. The discipline has seen the introduction of a number of adjuvant tools, including radiologic localizing studies and intraoperative parathyroid hormone (PTH) assays, which have dramatically impacted the ease and success rate of these operations. Consequently, particularly in experienced hands, greater than 95% of surgeries result in normocalcemia [2–4]. However, this leaves a small percentage of patients who are not cured with surgery or who go on to develop recurrent disease. Managing these patients can be challenging.

In contrast to primary parathyroid surgery, reoperative surgery has higher rates of complications and lower rates of success [5]. Due to scarring, loss of surgical planes, and distortion of normal anatomical positioning, detecting pathologic parathyroid glands in the remedial setting can be extremely arduous. Additionally, risk

M.C. Singer (✉)
Department of Otolaryngology – Head and Neck Surgery,
Division of Thyroid and Parathyroid Surgery, Henry Ford Health System,
2799 West Grand Blvd., Detroit, MI 48202, USA
e-mail: msinger1@hfhs.org

© Springer International Publishing AG 2018
R.P. Tufano, P.K. Pellitteri (eds.), *Reoperative Parathyroid Surgery*,
DOI 10.1007/978-3-319-60723-8_3

of injury to other structures, particularly the recurrent laryngeal nerve and normal parathyroid glands, is increased significantly. As a result, the risk-benefit profile for these cases must be carefully considered, and the decision to operate is not made as simply as in the primary setting.

Unfortunately, there are no clear established guidelines or list of indications for patients who are candidates for reoperative parathyroidectomy. This is due to the difficulty in easily categorizing these patients and the need to consider so many patient-specific variables in their care. Therefore, clinicians are left to determine the value of proceeding with reoperation on an individual case basis.

Debate exists among clinicians about the proper approach to reoperative parathyroidectomy. Some argue that the indications for remedial surgery are the same as for primary surgery. However, most believe that given the greater rates of complications and lower rates of success, a higher threshold must be met and multiple factors considered before proceeding with reoperation [6, 7].

Recurrent Versus Persistent Disease

After surgery, patients can demonstrate continued elevation of both serum calcium and PTH levels. Persistent hyperparathyroidism is defined by hypercalcemia that occurs within 6 months of initial surgery. This is in contrast to recurrent disease, whereby the patient experiences a period of eucalcemia that lasts at least 6 months. After this time, the patient's calcium levels again become elevated. Regardless of the designation, these patients are at risk for metabolic complications and associated symptoms of their disease.

Persistent disease is a result of unsuccessful initial surgery, with failure to find and excise the pathologic gland(s). Both persistent and recurrent disease can also be the result of inadequate resection of tissue in the setting of multiglandular disease, regrowth of pathologic tissue after subtotal resection, or growth of residual tissue after incomplete excision of an adenoma or carcinoma. Recurrent disease can also occur when pathologic tissue is seeded in the neck during initial surgery (i.e., parathyromatosis) or in the less common situation of de novo disease development in a previously non-pathologic gland.

Critically, patients with persistent or recurrent disease need to be differentiated from others who, after apparent curative surgery (based on intraoperative PTH levels), postoperatively achieve eucalcemia but demonstrate elevated PTH levels. This scenario has been reported to occur in up to 30% of patients undergoing what was felt to be successful parathyroidectomy [8]. An uninformed patient, surgeon, or referring physician may assume that this is a manifestation of persistent or recurrent disease. However, in these patients, the postoperative calcium levels are decreased prior to surgery and clearly within the normal range. Different theories have been proposed for this phenomenon, including that this is caused by subclinical bone hunger, a decreased peripheral sensitivity to PTH, or a relative vitamin D deficiency [9–12]. While a small percentage of these patients go on to develop frank recurrent disease, in most of these patients, the PTH levels eventually return to normal (with continued eucalcemia). This normalization occurs with increasing frequency as time passes after surgery. Reoperative surgery in these patients would be futile and inappropriate.

Confirm Diagnosis

In a patient with persistent or recurrent disease, prior to considering further intervention, the correct diagnosis must be made definitively. Even if a patient has previously been seen and a complete workup has already been performed, all relevant tests should be re-reviewed. Particularly, if a patient was previously managed by another physician (or institution), assumptions should not be made regarding the completeness of the assessment or the accuracy of the diagnosis.

Prior and repeat serum calcium, ionized calcium, PTH, 25-hydroxy vitamin D, and creatinine levels should be checked. If not previously performed, a 24 h urine collection should be completed. This can help rule out the possibility of familial hypocalciuric hypercalcemia (FHH), based on the fractional excretion of calcium (calcium/creatinine clearance ratio). If there is any question about the possibility of FHH being the true diagnosis, genetic testing can be obtained for CaSR mutation. Patients with FHH are not at risk of the sequelae of primary hyperparathyroidism and do not benefit from surgery.

Radiologic studies do not play a role in diagnosing primary hyperparathyroidism and should only be considered at the point when the diagnosis has already been confirmed and surgery is indicated.

Indications

While there is a general consensus about the indications for "first time" surgery in patients with primary hyperparathyroidism, some debate does exist, particularly in regard to "asymptomatic" patients. For patients who present with classical symptoms of primary hyperparathyroidism, such as nephrolithiasis, nephrocalcinosis, or osteitis fibrosa cystica, surgery should be performed.

However, this form of the disease is much less frequently encountered today. Much more commonly patients do not have the classical sequelae and are considered asymptomatic, though many have vague constitutional, musculoskeletal, or neurocognitive symptoms [13]. An expert panel of physicians, acting under the auspices of the National Institute of Health, has issued guidelines for surgical intervention in these asymptomatic patients [14–17]. These guidelines have gone through several iterations since 1990 but are widely utilized by physicians to direct patient care (Table 3.1).

Table 3.1 Current and previous recommended guidelines for surgery in patients with "asymptomatic" primary hyperparathyroidism

	1990	2002	2008	2013
Serum calcium (mg/dL above upper limit of normal)	1–1.6	1	1	1
Skeletal	DEXA z-score less than −2.0	DEXA t-score less than −2.5 at any site	1. DEXA t-score less than −2.5 at any site 2. History of fragility fracture	1. DEXA t-score less than −2.5 at lumbar spine, hip, femoral neck, or distal one third radius 2. Vertebral fracture
Renal	1. GFR reduced by more than 30% 2. 24 h urine calcium more than 400 mg/day	1. GFR reduced by more than 30% 2. 24 h urine calcium more than 400 mg/day	1. GFR less than 60 cc/min 2. 24 h urine calcium not recommended	1. GFR less than 60 cc/min 2. 24 h urine calcium more than 400 mg/day 3. Presence of nephrolithiasis or nephrocalcinosis
Age	<50 years	<50 years	<50 years	<50 years

No equivalent guidelines have been produced specifically for patients who might require reoperative parathyroidectomy. Consequently, in general, these same indications are appropriate to at least consider when contemplating the option of remedial surgery.

Decision to Proceed with Surgery

A confirmed diagnosis and proper indication are not a sufficient basis to proceed with reoperative parathyroidectomy. In fact, these two elements are the minimum threshold that must be established before surgery can even be considered.

When considering any medical treatment, the potential risks and benefits of said treatment modality need to be carefully weighed. With the excellent success rates and low incidence of complications in primary parathyroidectomy, making this assessment is often straightforward. However, as noted earlier, the likelihood of cure may be lower and the risk of complications possibly greater in reoperative parathyroidectomy. Therefore, for remedial surgery to be sensible, the strength of the indication and the related potential benefits should be greater in order to outweigh the increased risks.

Multiple factors impact the prospect for success without complication in reoperative parathyroidectomy. When considering surgery, the first step is to try to understand the cause of the persistent or recurrent disease. If it is the result of surgical failure, the reason for failure may be unclear. Anatomic, biologic, and/or surgical variables can be the basis for not achieving cure during initial surgery. In order to evaluate these potential variables, all prior notes, radiology examinations, operative reports, and pathology and lab results should be carefully reviewed. A major determinant in the success rate of reoperation is the number of glands responsible for the hyperparathyroidism. A single adenoma is more likely than multiglandular involvement to be successfully identified and excised during remedial surgery. Possible insight into the number of glands involved can be offered by lab results, imaging studies, family history, and operative findings, especially related to the extent of exploration. In regard to localization studies, simply examining radiology reports is never optimal when planning parathyroid surgery. However, in the context of remedial surgery, directly studying the images of these tests is absolutely essential. It is also paramount to understand which areas were dissected and examined and which may not have been; which parathyroid glands were removed, partially excised, or biopsied; and which gland(s) or remnant(s) were marked with clips or suture. It is wise to not accept as fact a surgeon's report of identifying a parathyroid gland(s) during surgery based on visualization alone.

Patient-specific elements then need to be assessed. Has the patient had prior thyroid surgery, anterior cervical disk fusion, or other neck operations? Is the patient's body habitus a potential obstacle because of difficulties it may cause with exposure? Does a high body mass index mean more extensive cervical fat and soft tissue, possibly a harbinger of a more challenging exploration? Are there signs of thyroiditis, which can lead to additional fibrosis, as well as extensive adenopathy (which may mimic pathologic parathyroid glands)?

When calculating the risk-benefit and success profile of possible reoperation, other patient factors that need consideration are the patient's age, occupation, lifestyle, and ability to tolerate potential complications and if they have had complications from the initial surgery that may make reoperative surgery even more dangerous. For example, based on career and lifestyle requirements, is a recurrent nerve injury going to be a simple inconvenience or a life-changing impediment? If a patient becomes temporarily or permanently hypocalcemic after surgery, are they going to be able to reliably take calcium and vitamin D supplements? These details should all be considered in potential reoperative patients.

Perhaps the most crucial determinant in deciding to proceed with reoperative surgery is the reliability of localization studies (discussed at length in separate chapter). Blind exploration in a previously operated field is extremely difficult and can lead to complications. Therefore, at many institutions, for the vast majority of patients who do not exhibit dramatic symptoms of the disease, the general approach is to only reoperate in the setting of well-localized disease [4, 18]. The results in these patients can be excellent, with success rates of reoperation of up to 95% when performed by an expert surgeon [19, 20].

In patients with severe metabolic complications, such as chronic nephrolithiasis or marked bone disease, there is a greater imperative to cure their hyperparathyroidism. Only in these patients should reoperative surgery without definitive localization be reasonably considered.

References

1. Giddings CE, Rimmer J, Weir N. History of parathyroid gland surgery: a historical case series. J Laryngol Otol. 2009;123:1075–81.
2. Allendorf J, DiGorgi M, Spanknebel K, et al. 1112 consecutive bilateral neck explorations for primary hyperparathyroidism. World J Surg. 2007;31:2075–80.
3. Clark OH. Symposium: parathyroid disease – part 1. Contemp Surg. 1998;52:137–52.
4. Jaskowiak N, Norton JA, Alexander HR, et al. A prospective trial evaluating a standard approach to reoperation for missed parathyroid adenoma. Ann Surg. 1996;224:308–20.
5. Shen W, Duren M, Morita E, et al. Reoperation for persistent or recurrent primary hyperparathyroidism. Arch Surg. 1996;131:861–7.
6. Prescott JD, Udelsman R. Remedial operation for primary hyperparathyroidism. World J Surg. 2009;22:2324–34.
7. Udelsman R. Approach to the patient with persistent or recurrent primary hyperparathyroidism. J Clin Endocrinol Metab. 2011;96:2950–8.
8. Oltman SC, Maalouf NM, Holt S. Significance of elevated parathyroid hormone after parathyroidectomy for primary hyperparathyroidism. Endocr Pract. 2011;17(suppl 1):57–62.
9. Carty SE, Roberts MM, Virji MA, et al. Elevated serum parathormone level after "concise parathyroidectomy" for primary sporadic hyperparathyroidism. Surgery. 2002;132:1086–92.
10. Ning L, Sippel R, Schaeger S, et al. What is the clinical significance of an elevated parathyroid hormone level after curative surgery for primary hyperparathyroidism. Ann Surg. 2009;249:469–72.
11. Westerdahl J, Valdemarsson S, Lindblom P, et al. Postoperative elevated serum levels of intact parathyroid hormone after surgery for parathyroid adenoma: sign of bone remineralization and decreased calcium absorption. World J Surg. 2000;24:1323–9.
12. Beyer TD, Solorzano CC, Prinz RA, et al. Oral vitamin D supplementation reduces the incidence of eucalcemic PTH elevation after surgery for primary hyperparathyroidism. Surgery. 2007;141:777–83.
13. Silverberg SJ, Clarke BL, Peacock M, et al. Current issues in the presentation of asymptomatic primary hyperparathyroidism: proceedings of the fourth international workshop. J Clin Endocrinol Metab. 2014;99:3580–94.
14. National Institutes of Health. Diagnosis and management of asymptomatic primary hyperparathyroidism: Consensus development conference. Consens Stat. 1990;8:1–18.
15. Bilezikian JP, Potts JT Jr, Fuleihan G-H, et al. Summary statement from a workshop on asymptomatic primary hyperparathyroidism: a perspective for the 21st century. J Clin Endocrinol Metab. 2002;87:5353–61.
16. Bilezikian JP, Khan AA, Potts JT Jr. Guidelines for the management of asymptomatic primary hyperparathyroidism: summary statement from the third international workshop. J Clin Endocrinol Metab. 2009;94:335–9.
17. Bilezikian JP, Brandi ML, Eastell R, et al. Guidelines for the management of asymptomatic primary hyperparathyroidism: summary statement from the fourth international workshop. J Clin Endocrinol Metab. 2014;99(10):3561–9.
18. Wells SA, Debenedetti MK, Doherty GM. Recurrent or persistent hyperparathyroidism. J Bone Miner Res. 2002;17:N158–62.
19. Udelsman R, Donovan PI. Remedial parathyroid surgery. Ann Surg. 2006;244:471–9.
20. Doherty GM, Weber B, Norton JA. Cost of unsuccessful surgery for primary hyperparathyroidism. Surgery. 1994;116:954–7.

Chapter 4
Reoperative Surgical Planning and Adjunct Localization Studies

Jonathon O. Russell, Salem I. Noureldine, Nafi Aygun, and Ralph P. Tufano

Introduction

Pathology of the parathyroid glands is fairly prevalent in the United States. Each year, approximately ten cases of primary hyperparathyroidism (HPT) per 100,000 people are diagnosed in those younger than 40 years. The incidence is estimated to be four times higher in patients older than 60 years of age [1]. Surgery for primary HPT, performed by an experienced surgeon, is curative in more than 95% of cases [2]. In contrast, the success rate for low-volume surgeons is only 70% [3]. Consequently, the hyperparathyroid state may not be cured for a number of patients following surgery. Those not cured either remain hypercalcemic in the immediate postoperative period or redevelop hypercalcemia after a period of normocalcemia. Hypercalcemia persisting or recurring within 6 months after initial parathyroidectomy is referred to as *persistent HPT*. Hypercalcemia recurring more than 6 months after an apparently curative initial parathyroidectomy is referred to as *recurrent HPT*. Regardless of terminology, in both cases, the patient is at continued risk of metabolic complications from hypercalcemia and may continue to have discomfort from the associated symptoms. Despite advances in preoperative imaging and adjunctive intraoperative tools, the incidence of persistent or recurrent HPT has been reported to be as high as 30% [4–6].

J.O. Russell • S.I. Noureldine • R.P. Tufano (✉)
Department of Otolaryngology – Head and Neck Surgery, Johns Hopkins School
of Medicine, 601 N. Caroline St., Baltimore, MD 21287, USA
e-mail: rtufano@jhmi.edu

N. Aygun
Radiology and Radiological Science-Neuroradiology, Department of Radiology,
Johns Hopkins Medical Institutions, 601 N. Caroline St., Baltimore, MD 21287, USA

© Springer International Publishing AG 2018
R.P. Tufano, P.K. Pellitteri (eds.), *Reoperative Parathyroid Surgery*,
DOI 10.1007/978-3-319-60723-8_4

The indications for surgical intervention in reoperative cases must be clear, because the morbidity and technical difficulty are increased. Reoperations are unfortunately associated with a lower success rate than initial operations. Nonetheless, in experienced hands, the success rate of reoperative parathyroidectomy for persistent and recurrent HPT is reported to be more than 80–90% [7]. However, the ideal period to cure the patient is during the initial operation, when the risks of surgical complications are least likely and the likelihood of cure is greatest. This chapter aims to outline a perioperative scheme for approaching persistent and recurrent primary HPT.

Evaluation

It has been estimated that 2–10% of surgical failures may be attributed to an incorrect preoperative diagnosis of primary HPT [8, 9]. Accordingly, one of the key requirements for success in reoperative parathyroidectomy is a proper diagnosis. The initial step is to perform a thorough personal and family history for endocrine diseases and a physical examination. The history should be focused on ruling out differential diagnoses. By definition, HPT (primary or secondary) must be confirmed with an elevated serum calcium concentration and an elevated or inappropriately high serum parathyroid hormone (PTH) level. Patients may also present with elevated serum PTH and serum calcium levels at the upper limit of normal (the so-called normocalcemic hyperparathyroidism). Checking an ionized calcium level can help confirm the diagnosis of HPT in most of these patients. Elevated serum chloride and decreased serum phosphate levels are frequently noted. In addition, if not previously performed, benign familial hypocalciuric hypercalcemia should be ruled out with an appropriately elevated 24 h urinary calcium measurement and subsequent genetic testing if indicated. If all these parameters are not present, other causes of hypercalcemia must be considered (i.e., patients with normocalcemic HPT caused by hypoalbuminemia, hyperphosphatemia, vitamin D deficiency, or hypomagnesemia), because a repeat parathyroidectomy is almost guaranteed to be unrewarding in these circumstances. The diagnosis of HPT has been facilitated by the development of immunometric assays [10, 11]. Clinical analysis with immunometric PTH assays typically distinguishes hypercalcemic patients with HPT from patients with other causes of hypercalcemia. Diagnostic errors of hyperparathyroidism can result from medications (i.e., calcium, vitamin D, furosemide, thiazide diuretics, calcitonin, or lithium), malignancy (i.e., bone metastases or humoral hypercalcemia), granulomatous disease (i.e. sarcoidosis), acute renal failure, bone disease (i.e., Paget's disease or immobilization), hyperthyroidism, or adrenal insufficiency. Given the complexity of alternative explanations, a close relationship with medical specialists including endocrinologists can be invaluable to ensure that consensus is reached before the decision for further intervention is made. Such a relationship is likewise imperative in situations of more virulent forms of HPT, such as MEN, where multigland removal may be necessary.

With a confirmed diagnosis of persistent or recurrent HPT, further information obtained by clinical evaluation, review of preoperative localization studies, operative reports, and pathology reports is critical to help determine the location of potentially normal and abnormal glands. The operative report should document the extent of the initial parathyroidectomy; which parathyroid glands were identified; whether these glands were excised, biopsied, and/or clipped to mark for future identification; where scar tissue can be expected to be encountered; the relationship of the glands to the recurrent laryngeal nerve; intraoperative PTH results if evaluated; and the number and the position of normal and abnormal glands. Unfortunately, it often doesn't contain most of these components which are all critical to operative planning. The pathology report confirms how many parathyroid glands were indeed excised, whether biopsied glands were definitely parathyroid tissue, and whether parathyroid glands examined were normal or hypercellular. Review of old pathology slides may be required. It may be useful to correlate previous localization studies with intraoperative findings. Direct laryngoscopy is necessary before reoperation to assess vocal fold function.

Localization Studies

A battery of localization studies prior to reoperation are usually employed, due to the associated risks of surgical complications and the lower likelihood of surgical cure. Approximately 90% of missed parathyroid tumors can be removed through the initial cervical incision. Successful localization permits a focused approach in most cases. This limits the amount of dissection required, preferably to a unilateral approach, as one prefers not to perform bilateral re-exploration when possible, avoiding the increased risk of hypoparathyroidism and RLN injury [12, 13]. Localization studies, in combination with previous information from operative and histologic findings, usually direct the surgeon to the abnormal parathyroid gland, thus minimizing complications and shortening the operative time. Knowledge of anatomy and expected locations of both normal and ectopic locations for parathyroid glands is paramount in reoperative parathyroidectomy, and the reader is referred to previous chapters. A variety of invasive and noninvasive techniques are available to image or localize abnormal parathyroid glands. Intraoperative PTH monitoring is a helpful adjunct for confirming when all abnormal parathyroid tissue has been removed [14–17].

Non-Invasive Methods

As in the initial work up of primary HPT, a number of imaging studies are available for the evaluation of recurrent or persistent HPT. Unfortunately, all available imaging modalities are far from perfect, and it is common practice to obtain multiple studies in this setting as the accuracy of two concordant exams is higher than a single localizing exam [18]. Despite all efforts, there can be a high rate of nonlocalization which requires further workup with invasive tests. The abnormal parathyroid glands are mostly found in eutopic locations although there are higher rates of mediastinal, intrathyroid, and intrathymic glands as well as multigland disease in the reoperative setting. Local expertise and availability of imaging technology are the most important factors in determining which imaging algorithm is followed [19, 20].

Ultrasound (US)

Ultrasound's sensitivity is quite low given the potentially increased incidence of mediastinal glands in a reoperative scenario, and the inability to visualize with US. However, the majority of abnormal glands are in eutopic locations, and US remains the most cost-effective and least harmful imaging study to start with, as it does not involve radiation exposure or contrast administration.

Multiphase CT

Most centers perform an unenhanced CT followed by one, two, or three additional acquisitions after intravenous contrast administration. CT takes advantage of the fact that parathyroid glands are more vascular compared to the surrounding tissue and show a greater degree of enhancement in the arterial phase of the acquisition followed by a sharp decrease in attenuation in the venous phase due to rapid wash-out. In addition, state-of-the-art CT exams provide exquisite anatomic detail. When an abnormal gland is confidently identified with multiphase CT, surgical eligibility can be confirmed even if US and sestamibi scans are nonlocalizing [21, 22]. It has been demonstrated that two phases may be sufficient, thus sparing the patient additional ionizing radiation [23]. Intrathyroid adenomas are relatively difficult to localize with CT as arterial enhancement and venous washout features of adenomas and the thyroid gland nodules are often similar.

MRI

MRI is not commonly utilized outside a few centers in localizing abnormal parathyroid glands. Multiparametric imaging and high contrast resolution provides a greater ability to differentiate adenomas from the surrounding tissue. Dynamic contrast-enhanced sequences allow assessment of blood flow through parathyroid glands in a similar fashion with multiphase CT and increase MRI's accuracy compared to standard protocols [24].

Sestamibi Scan

Because Tc sestamibi is accumulated and retained by the mitochondria-rich oxyphil cells in parathyroid glands more than thyroid tissue, it is more specific compared to other imaging modalities, although its sensitivity is limited due to lower spatial resolution. Thus, it often fails to localize small glands. SPECT is an acquisition technique that affords higher sensitivity and anatomic accuracy compared to planar Tc sestamibi scans. When SPECT is combined with other modalities in multiphase fusion techniques such as SPECT/CT, localization is further improved [25].

Invasive Methods

Fine needle aspiration biopsy may be applied using both computed tomographic and ultrasound guidance for correct needle placement in suspected abnormal parathyroid tissue during localization in preparation for reoperative surgery. Investigations have shown FNA to be a specific modality in distinguishing between parathyroid and nonparathyroid tissues [26, 27]. Cytologic evaluation of tissue samples obtained by fine needle aspiration biopsy is less sensitive than measuring washout PTH levels of the aspirate material, because follicular thyroid tumors may be misinterpreted as parathyroid tissue under cytologic review. The role of FNA in reoperative parathyroid surgery can be especially helpful in situations where a thyroid nodule is noted and imaging is suggestive of a possible intrathyroidal parathyroid adenoma, which is otherwise rare. It may also be particularly helpful in a multiply operated patient where there is intense scarring and a focused surgery would be most prudent.

Selective Arteriography

Selective angiographic injection of the inferior thyroid arteries will demonstrate a vascular blush which may be present in up to 25–70% of parathyroid adenomas [28]. Although rare, significant complications attributable to this technique have been reported and include central nervous system embolic infarction and potential quadriplegia [29]. As a consequence of these potential risks and because of improvements in noninvasive imaging studies, selective parathyroid arteriography is rarely performed and should be reserved for patients who need surgery and in whom previous noninvasive testing has failed to identify the adenoma in a usual or ectopic location [29].

Selective Venous Sampling

Similar to super-selective digital subtraction angiography, selective venous sampling is reserved for selected patients. This modality is performed by catheterization of veins draining the neck and mediastinum [30]. By obtaining blood samples and comparing PTH levels obtained from sampling of the iliac veins with those obtained from thyroid veins (superior, middle, and inferior), vertebral veins, and the thymic vein, the anticipated localization of the adenoma will be within the area where venous PTH levels are at least twice as high as the systemic levels. Selective venous sampling has been shown to be more accurate than large vein sampling, with accuracy of 83% as contrasted to 29%, respectively [30]. This modality became significantly more accurate with the utilization of improved intact parathyroid hormone (iPTH) assays, which increased the sensitivity of venous sampling to 87–95% in some investigations [31]. Selective venous sampling should be reserved for patients requiring reoperation and in whom noninvasive studies are negative, equivocal, or conflicting. This modality is technically challenging, and its success depends on an experienced interventional radiologist [32].

Intraoperative Adjuncts

Intraoperative US

The availability of high-resolution US has led some surgeons to further utilize it in their operating room. Intraoperative US may be useful in a number of operative settings, primarily that of re-exploration in a neck that demonstrates significant surgical fibrosis. Using this adjunct will allow one to scan the neck and, where possible, correlate structures with preoperative images just prior to surgery. This achieves accurate visualization of the ultimate position of both the parathyroid lesion and other structures in the neck, in particular the relation to the internal jugular vein and carotid artery. This technique may also assist in precisely localizing the incision once the patient is in the neck extension position, for an ideal access for removal of parathyroid tissue. US can be combined with fine needle aspiration for PTH to interrogate hypoechoic structures identified in the thyroid or neck intraoperatively. Utilization of US once surgical exploration begins is compromised by disruption of tissue planes and is not often helpful.

Methylene Blue Injection

In rare circumstances, methylene blue has been used by some surgeons in reoperative settings, due to the dye's ability to preferentially stain the parathyroid glands when perioperative adjuncts have been misleading. The rationale for using methylene blue is to facilitate correct parathyroid gland identification and thus minimize the complication rate [33, 34]. Unfortunately, the literature is plagued with growing numbers of reports describing significant side effects to its use such as encephalopathy or central nervous system toxicity, as well as specific interaction with serotonin reuptake inhibitors causing severe cardiovascular changes and neurological dysfunction [33, 35–37]. Furthermore, intraoperative changes to pulse oximetry readings can be problematic for anesthesiologists. Because of these precautions and the little added value, methylene blue is not routinely used and should not be routinely utilized for intraoperative identification of parathyroid tissue.

Gamma Probe

Tc-99 m sestamibi uptake by parathyroid tissue is a function of metabolic activity. This forms the basis for utilizing sestamibi scans to localize hypersecreting parathyroid glands in patients with primary HPT. Patients are injected with a Tc-99 m sestamibi isotope on the day of surgery, usually within approximately 2 h of the operation. A handheld gamma probe is used to direct the incision site and to localize the abnormal parathyroid glands. The initial scan provides information regarding localization of presumed adenomas and the presence of delayed uptake of nuclear material within the thyroid gland. After identification and removal of the abnormal parathyroid gland, the gamma probe may be used to confirm high metabolic activity within the resected tissue as compared with the radioactivity of the surgical bed, thus validating that no additional hyperactive glands remain behind. Potential advantages of radioguided parathyroid identification include facilitation of targeted parathyroidectomy, shorter operating time, and verification of successful surgery. Absolute contraindications for radioguided parathyroidectomy include pregnancy and allergy or sensitivity to Tc-99 m sestamibi. The 20-percent rule, published by Murphy and Norman [38], suggests that any excised tissue containing more than 20% of background radioactivity in a patient with a positive sestamibi scan is consistent with the finding of a solitary parathyroid adenoma. This protocol, however, has limited ability to exclude nonparathyroid tissue or multiglandular disease, and the signal is proportional to the gland size [39–42].

The overall accuracy of radioguided parathyroidectomy is 83% with a conversion rate to bilateral neck exploration of 10% for single-gland disease, 50% for multiglandular disease, and 50% for hyperplasia [41, 43]. The gamma probe is considered unhelpful in up to 48% of cases [40, 44]. The limitations include logistic difficulties with timing isotope injection, equipment problems, confusing counts, and easily identified abnormal glands. Therefore, most parathyroid surgeons will only consider intraoperative radioguided parathyroidectomy in patients with ectopic parathyroid adenoma or previous thyroidectomy where confusing background counts are not a concern. If concerned about persistent uptake of nuclear material by the thyroid, thyroid suppression may be accomplished preoperatively in order to minimize background counts which can obscure identification of the targeted parathyroid gland.

Frozen Section Analysis

The histological identification of parathyroid tissue relies on the identification of three types of cells that comprise the parathyroid tissue: (1) chief, (2) oxyphil, and (3) water clear cells. Chief cells are similar to thyroid follicular cells, and oxyphil cells are indistinguishable from thyroid Hurthle cells; thus, the distinction of parathyroid from thyroid tissue is more challenging. However, follicles and colloid-like material are uncommon in parathyroid specimens. Despite limitations, the use of frozen section to distinguish parathyroid tissue from nonparathyroid tissue has an accuracy of 99.2% [45].

Frozen section is an unreliable method for distinguishing between multiglandular disease and adenomas [46]. The distinction between hyperplasia and adenoma is not based on pathologic criteria, but rather on the operative findings. If the pathologist receives a biopsy from a single parathyroid gland for frozen section interpretation, a possible diagnosis would be hypercellular parathyroid tissue. An adenoma can only be diagnosed with confidence if only one gland of the four glands is enlarged and hypercellular. Therefore, without biopsies from all four glands, the pathologist is unable to determine the cellular constituency of the remaining parathyroid glands and definitively suggest that a gland is a parathyroid adenoma.

There is also a role for frozen section in subtotal or total parathyroidectomy for multigland disease and secondary and tertiary hyperparathyroidism. In these cases, the surgeon may choose cryopreservation or implantation of parathyroid tissue. The use of frozen section is more common in these situations to positively diagnose parathyroid tissue prior to implantation.

Needless to say, documentation of prior removal of four normal parathyroid glands is very worrisome for a missed supernumerary parathyroid adenoma. Failure to perform autotransplantation of parathyroid tissue following removal of any remaining parathyroid tissue would likely result in permanent hypoparathyroidism. This underscores the need to thoroughly evaluate both the prior operative and pathology reports and to discuss the case directly with the surgeons involved in the prior operations where discrepancy exists.

IOPTH

To further improve the surgical success of targeted parathyroidectomy and to minimize the possibility of persistent or recurrent hyperparathyroidism after surgery, some have advocated for the use of surgical adjuncts such as IOPTH monitoring. In 1990, Dr. George Irvin of the University of Miami revolutionized parathyroid surgery by measuring IOPTH levels and confirming removal of hypersecreting parathyroid glands. IOPTH is useful in assessing the adequacy of resection by functional means without the need to expose all the parathyroid glands. Before exiting the operating room, the surgeon can feel confident that the patient will most likely be eucalcemic by demonstrating an appropriate reduction in IOPTH levels after excision of all hyperfunctioning parathyroid tissue. The ability to confirm complete removal of all hypersecreting glands and predict operative success minimizes operative time, diminishes the need for bilateral neck exploration, and improves cure rates [14]. IOPTH is based on the short half-life of circulating PTH. PTH is cleared from the blood in an early rapid phase with a half-life variously reported as 1.5–21.5 min in patients with normal renal function. PTH levels are measured preoperatively and at set post-excision times. Due to the different IOPTH decrease criteria for a successful operation, several studies aimed to identify the optimal criteria and predictive cure rate. A decline of more than 50% in PTH level from the highest pre-incision or pre-excision level is associated with a predictive cure in 94–97% of cases [15–17]. We prefer a PTH drop of more than 50% and into the normal range before concluding the procedure [16, 47]. The use of IOPTH is recommended for patients undergoing targeted parathyroidectomy. Different criteria may be utilized with similar accuracy rates. When used correctly, we believe that IOPTH is the most accurate adjunct to predict eucalcemia available to the surgeon performing parathyroid surgery.

Conclusion

Reoperative parathyroidectomy can be challenging to even the most experienced parathyroid surgeon. Successful reoperation demands preoperative collaboration from the fields of endocrinology, radiology, and surgery. Attention to detail with the appropriate invasive and noninvasive imaging modalities is necessary for consistent outcomes. Intraoperative adjuncts, while helpful, may not compensate for inadequate preoperative planning.

References

1. Heath H III, Hodgson SF, Kennedy MA. Primary hyperparathyroidism. Incidence, morbidity, and potential economic impact in a community. N Engl J Med. 1980;302(4):189–93.
2. Clark OH. Symposium: parathyroid disease—part 1. Contemp Surg. 1998;52:137–52.
3. Malmaeus J, Granberg PO, Halvorsen J, Akerstrom G, Johansson H. Parathyroid surgery in Scandinavia. Acta Chir Scand. 1988;154(7–8):409–13.
4. Wadstrom C, Zedenius J, Guinea A, Reeve TS, Delbridge L. Re-operative surgery for recurrent or persistent primary hyperparathyroidism. Aust N Z J Surg. 1998;68(2):103–7.
5. Mundschenk J, Klose S, Lorenz K, Dralle H, Lehnert H. Diagnostic strategies and surgical procedures in persistent or recurrent primary hyperparathyroidism. Exp Clin Endocrinol Diabetes. 1999;107(6):331–6.
6. Al-Fehaily M, Clark OH. Persistent or recurrent primary hyperparathyroidism. Ann Ital Chir. 2003;74(4):423–34.
7. Caron NR, Sturgeon C, Clark OH. Persistent and recurrent hyperparathyroidism. Curr Treat Options in Oncol. 2004;5(4):335–45.
8. Clark OH, Way LW, Hunt TK. Recurrent hyperparathyroidism. Ann Surg. 1976;184(4):391–402.
9. Marx SJ, Stock JL, Attie MF, Downs RW Jr, Gardner DG, Brown EM, et al. Familial hypocalciuric hypercalcemia: recognition among patients referred after unsuccessful parathyroid exploration. Ann Intern Med. 1980;92(3):351–6.
10. Brown RC, Aston JP, Weeks I, Woodhead JS. Circulating intact parathyroid hormone measured by a two-site immunochemiluminometric assay. J Clin Endocrinol Metab. 1987;65(3):407–14.
11. Bouillon R, Coopmans W, Degroote DE, Radoux D, Eliard PH. Immunoradiometric assay of parathyrin with polyclonal and monoclonal region-specific antibodies. Clin Chem. 1990;36(2):271–6.
12. Wells SA Jr, Debenedetti MK, Doherty GM. Recurrent or persistent hyperparathyroidism. J Bone Miner Res. 2002;17(Suppl 2):N158–62.

13. Mariette C, Pellissier L, Combemale F, Quievreux JL, Carnaille B, Proye C. Reoperation for persistent or recurrent primary hyperparathyroidism. Langenbeck's Arch Surg. 1998;383(2):174–9.
14. Chen H, Pruhs Z, Starling JR, Mack E. Intraoperative parathyroid hormone testing improves cure rates in patients undergoing minimally invasive parathyroidectomy. Surgery. 2005;138(4):583–7. discussion 7–90
15. Carneiro DM, Solorzano CC, Nader MC, Ramirez M, Irvin GL III. Comparison of intraoperative iPTH assay (QPTH) criteria in guiding parathyroidectomy: which criterion is the most accurate? Surgery. 2003;134(6):973–9. discussion 9–81
16. Chiu B, Sturgeon C, Angelos P. Which intraoperative parathyroid hormone assay criterion best predicts operative success? A study of 352 consecutive patients. Arch Surg. 2006;141(5):483–7. discussion 7–8
17. Irvin GL III, Solorzano CC, Carneiro DM. Quick intraoperative parathyroid hormone assay: surgical adjunct to allow limited parathyroidectomy, improve success rate, and predict outcome. World J Surg. 2004;28(12):1287–92.
18. Kutler DI, Moquete R, Kazam E, Kuhel WI. Parathyroid localization with modified 4D-computed tomography and ultrasonography for patients with primary hyperparathyroidism. Laryngoscope. 2011;121(6):1219–24.
19. McIntyre CJ, Allen JL, Constantinides VA, Jackson JE, Tolley NS, Palazzo FF. Patterns of disease in patients at a tertiary referral centre requiring reoperative parathyroidectomy. Ann R Coll Surg Engl. 2015;97(8):598–602.
20. Parikh PP, Farra JC, Allan BJ, Lew JI. Long-term effectiveness of localization studies and intraoperative parathormone monitoring in patients undergoing reoperative parathyroidectomy for persistent or recurrent hyperparathyroidism. Am J Surg. 2015;210(1):117–22.
21. Ginsburg M, Christoforidis GA, Zivin SP, Obara P, Wroblewski K, Angelos P, et al. Adenoma localization for recurrent or persistent primary hyperparathyroidism using dynamic four-dimensional CT and venous sampling. J Vasc Interv Radiol. 2015;26(1):79–86.
22. Cham S, Sepahdari AR, Hall KE, Yeh MW, Harari A. Dynamic parathyroid computed tomography (4DCT) facilitates reoperative parathyroidectomy and enables cure of missed hyperplasia. Ann Surg Oncol. 2015;22(11):3537–42.
23. Noureldine SI, Aygun N, Walden MJ, Hassoon A, Gujar SK, Tufano RP. Multiphase computed tomography for localization of parathyroid disease in patients with primary hyperparathyroidism: how many phases do we really need? Surgery. 2014;156(6):1300–6. discussion 13006–7
24. Kluijfhout WP, Venkatesh S, Beninato T, Vriens MR, Duh QY, Wilson DM, et al. Performance of magnetic resonance imaging in the evaluation of first-time and reoperative primary hyperparathyroidism. Surgery. 2016;160(3):747–54.
25. Lavely WC, Goetze S, Friedman KP, Leal JP, Zhang Z, Garret-Mayer E, et al. Comparison of SPECT/CT, SPECT, and planar imaging with single- and dual-phase (99m)Tc-sestamibi parathyroid scintigraphy. J Nucl Med. 2007;48(7):1084–9.
26. MacFarlane MP, Fraker DL, Shawker TH, Norton JA, Doppman JL, Chang RA, et al. Use of preoperative fine-needle aspiration in patients undergoing reoperation for primary hyperparathyroidism. Surgery. 1994;116(6):959–64. discussion 64–5
27. Stephen AE, Milas M, Garner CN, Wagner KE, Siperstein AE. Use of surgeon-performed office ultrasound and parathyroid fine needle aspiration for complex parathyroid localization. Surgery. 2005;138(6):1143–50. discussion 50–1
28. Sachs BA, Pollatta J. Angiographic ablation of parathyroid adenomas. In: Kadir S, editor. Current practice of interventional radiology. Philadelphia, PA: BC Decker; 1991.
29. Miller DL, Chang R, Doppman JL, Norton JA. Localization of parathyroid adenomas: superselective arterial DSA versus superselective conventional angiography. Radiology. 1989;170(3 Pt 2):1003–6.
30. Sugg SL, Fraker DL, Alexander R, Doppman JL, Miller DL, Chang R, et al. Prospective evaluation of selective venous sampling for parathyroid hormone concentration in patients undergoing reoperations for primary hyperparathyroidism. Surgery. 1993;114(6):1004–9. discussion 9–10

31. Jones JJ, Brunaud L, Dowd CF, Duh QY, Morita E, Clark OH. Accuracy of selective venous sampling for intact parathyroid hormone in difficult patients with recurrent or persistent hyperparathyroidism. Surgery. 2002;132(6):944–50. discussion 50–1

32. Lebastchi AH, Aruny JE, Donovan PI, Quinn CE, Callender GG, Carling T, et al. Real-time super selective venous sampling in remedial parathyroid surgery. J Am Coll Surg. 2015;220(6):994–1000.

33. Pollack G, Pollack A, Delfiner J, Fernandez J. Parathyroid surgery and methylene blue: a review with guidelines for safe intraoperative use. Laryngoscope. 2009;119(10):1941–6.

34. Kuriloff DB, Sanborn KV. Rapid intraoperative localization of parathyroid glands utilizing methylene blue infusion. Otolaryngol Head Neck Surg. 2004;131(5):616–22.

35. Han N, Bumpous JM, Goldstein RE, Fleming MM, Flynn MB. Intra-operative parathyroid identification using methylene blue in parathyroid surgery. Am Surg. 2007;73(8):820–3.

36. Ahmed TS. Methylene blue toxicity following infusion to localize parathyroid adenoma. J Laryngol Otol. 2006;120:708. author reply -9

37. Vutskits L, Briner A, Klauser P, Gascon E, Dayer AG, Kiss JZ, et al. Adverse effects of methylene blue on the central nervous system. Anesthesiology. 2008;108(4):684–92.

38. Murphy C, Norman J. The 20% rule: a simple, instantaneous radioactivity measurement defines cure and allows elimination of frozen sections and hormone assays during parathyroidectomy. Surgery. 1999;126(6):1023–8. discussion 8–9

39. Rubello D, Casara D, Giannini S, Piotto A, De Carlo E, Muzzio PC, et al. Importance of radio-guided minimally invasive parathyroidectomy using hand-held gamma probe and low (99m)Tc-MIBI dose. Technical considerations and long-term clinical results. Q J Nucl Med. 2003;47(2):129–38.

40. Jaskowiak NT, Sugg SL, Helke J, Koka MR, Kaplan EL. Pitfalls of intraoperative quick parathyroid hormone monitoring and gamma probe localization in surgery for primary hyperparathyroidism. Arch Surg. 2002;137(6):659–68. discussion 68–9

41. Chen H, Mack E, Starling JR. Radioguided parathyroidectomy is equally effective for both adenomatous and hyperplastic glands. Ann Surg. 2003;238(3):332–7. discussion 7–8

42. Ugur O, Bozkurt MF, Hamaloglu E, Sokmensuer C, Etikan I, Ugur Y, et al. Clinicopathologic and radiopharmacokinetic factors affecting gamma probe-guided parathyroidectomy. Arch Surg. 2004;139(11):1175–9.

43. Chen H, Mack E, Starling JR. A comprehensive evaluation of perioperative adjuncts during minimally invasive parathyroidectomy: which is most reliable? Ann Surg. 2005;242(3):375–80. discussion 80–3

44. Inabnet WB III, Kim CK, Haber RS, Lopchinsky RA. Radioguidance is not necessary during parathyroidectomy. Arch Surg. 2002;137(8):967–70.

45. Westra WH, Pritchett DD, Udelsman R. Intraoperative confirmation of parathyroid tissue during parathyroid exploration: a retrospective evaluation of the frozen section. Am J Surg Pathol. 1998;22(5):538–44.

46. Hosking SW, Jones H, du Boulay CE, McGinn FP. Surgery for parathyroid adenoma and hyperplasia: relationship of histology to outcome. Head Neck. 1993;15(1):24–8.

47. Clerici T, Brandle M, Lange J, Doherty GM, Gauger PG. Impact of intraoperative parathyroid hormone monitoring on the prediction of multiglandular parathyroid disease. World J Surg. 2004;28(2):187–92.

Chapter 5
Surgical Algorithm for Recurrent and Peristent Hyperparathyroidism

Phillip K. Pellitteri

Introduction

Persistent and recurrent hyperparathyroidism occurs in approximately 3.2% and 0.7% of patients, respectively. Taken together, these circumstances may be termed recalcitrant hyperparathyroidism. Initial studies of patients with persistent or recurrent elevated calcium levels after an initial parathyroid procedure suggested that the majority of patients in this category had multiglandular disease not appreciated at the initial operation [1–3]. However, these reports originated from institutional series with considerable experience in parathyroid surgery and are not representative of the general population after a failed parathyroid procedure [4]. A missed single abnormal parathyroid adenoma accounts for the majority of patients who fail initial procedures for the treatment of primary hyperparathyroidism [5, 6]. The causes for failed cervical exploration include the presence of multiple abnormal, ectopic, or supernumerary glands, surgeon experience, inadequate exploration of the neck and superior mediastinum, and incomplete resection of hyperplastic glands [4, 7]. Those patients not cured by the first operation pose a significant problem because of the more difficult and technically demanding nature of re-operative parathyroid surgery. As a result of scarring and distortion of normal tissue planes in the neck after a prior cervical exploration, success rates at subsequent surgery for primary hyperparathyroidism are decreased, and operative complications, including recurrent laryngeal nerve injury with vocal cord paralysis and hypoparathyroidism, can be even more problematic.

P.K. Pellitteri (✉)
Department of Otolaryngology/Head and Neck Surgery, Guthrie Health System,
One Guthrie Square, Sayre, PA 18840, USA
e-mail: phillip.pellitteri@guthrie.org

© Springer International Publishing AG 2018

R.P. Tufano, P.K. Pellitteri (eds.), *Reoperative Parathyroid Surgery*,
DOI 10.1007/978-3-319-60723-8_5

Operative Strategy

Following the decision to proceed with re-exploration and having performed a review of the initial operative procedure and localization studies, the surgeon then considers the operative approach. Ideally, the objective is to remove a single gland without extensive dissection, which may result in injury to the surrounding structures, i.e., recurrent laryngeal nerve or devascularization of remaining parathyroid tissue. The likelihood of accomplishing the objective is very dependent upon two factors: the experience of the initial operating surgeon and the demonstration of an enlarged hyperfunctional parathyroid gland on correlative localization studies.

In most cases, reoperation following initial surgery by an experienced surgeon will be difficult and tedious because the initial dissection that will have been comprehensive and the surgical bed will have significant fibrosis. In contradistinction, the extensiveness of initial exploration and resulting degree of fibrosis may be significantly less in patients having had the original surgery performed by a relatively inexperienced surgeon. In both of these circumstances, a localizing study will be of prime importance in targeting the putative hyperfunctional gland and limiting the re-operative dissection.

The best of all scenarios, and the most common, is unequivocal localization to a cervical site, which may also include the anterior superior mediastinum. The previous neck incision is generally used for access, in some cases by excising the old scar completely. The usual superior/inferior flaps are raised and access gained to the side of the neck indicated by the localization studies. A lateral to medial approach to dissection is undertaken, to avoid the dense fibrosis in the region of the tracheoesophageal groove where the recurrent laryngeal nerve resides. In this manner, dissection proceeds medially from the sternocleidomastoid muscle superficial to the great vessels and then directly to the region overlying the cervical spine. This approach exploits the concept of the viscero-vertebral angle (VVA), as described by Tenta [8]. This potential anatomic space is defined as that area bordered laterally by the carotid sheath structures, medially by the trachea and esophagus, anteriorly by the thyroid, and posteriorly by the cervical spine (Fig. 5.1). In accessing this region, the surgeon may take advantage of a tissue plane with relatively little vascularity and fibrosis. This area will allow extension to examine the superior mediastinum inferiorly, the retroesophageal compartment medially, and as far as the hyoid bone superiorly, all within planes of dissection that separate with relative freedom. The recurrent laryngeal nerve may be identified and extensively exposed for protection during this approach. Dense fibrosis is infrequently encountered over the prevertebral space, even following a thorough initial exploration. In the event a gland is suspected in the superior retro-thyroidal area, the nerve should be identified as it may be lateral to a medially displaced superior gland. The majority of missed adenomas, which are accessible through a cervical incision, may be approached using this technique, which also allows for thyroidectomy if necessary. A situation whereby localization studies indicate a mediastinal location usually mandates a thoracic approach, either by median sternotomy or lateral open or video-assisted thoracotomy, depending on the location within the mediasti-

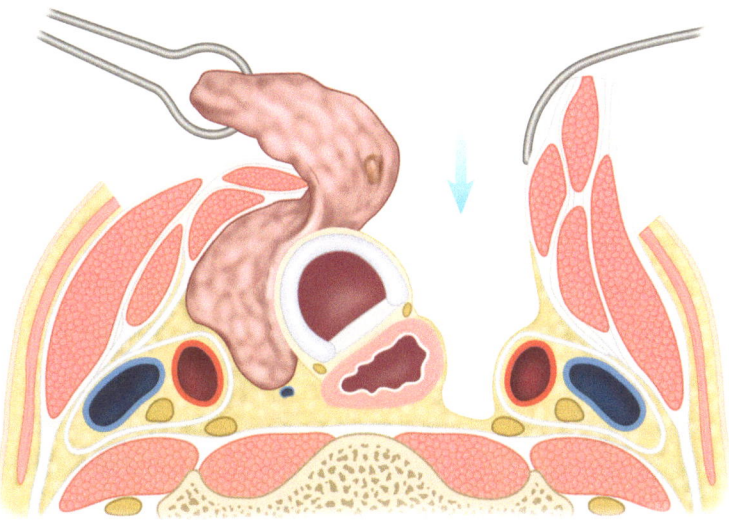

Fig. 5.1   The viscero-vertebral angle approach

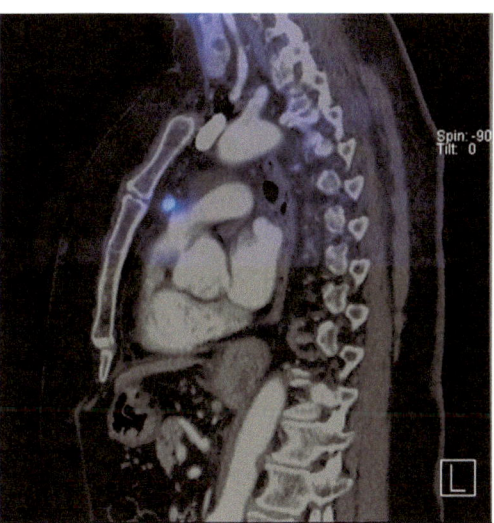

Fig. 5.2   Mediastinal parathyroid adenoma within middle posterior compartment demonstrated in fusion imaging

num. An enlarged gland identified within the anterior mediastinum and not accessible transcervically is usually associated with the thymus and may be accessed by either median sternotomy or video-assisted mediastinoscopy. These glands are usually found at the level of the innominate vein within thymic tissue but may also be found adjacent to the aortic arch or between the thymus and pleura. Should the localization studies demonstrate a posterior-based mediastinal gland, a lateral or posterolateral approach should be undertaken, either with open or video-assisted (VATS) technique

Fig. 5.3 Thoracoscopic
approach to mediastinal
parathyroid adenoma
shown in Fig. 5.2

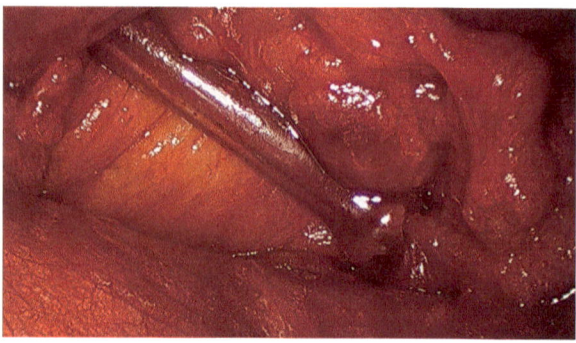

(Figs. 5.2 and 5.3) in order to avoid dissection thru critical structures in the anterior
mediastinum. These posterior-based glands may reside in the aortopulmonary window or the retroesophageal region. One should be aware that the recurrent laryngeal
nerve may be injured when approaching the posterior mediastinum through a left
lateral thoracotomy. Despite what may be interpreted as compelling localization
results, the surgeon should be prepared to perform concurrent cervical exploration in
the event that initial intra-operative PTH levels (IOPTH) do not confirm removal of all
hyperfunctional parathyroid tissue.

The most problematic preoperative scenario to confront is that in which localization fails to identify any suspicious putative site suggestive of parathyroid abnormality. It is in this situation where re-operative surgery for hyperparathyroidism is
potentially the least successful and the most morbid. Failure to localize usually
mandates a bilateral cervical exploration that comprehensively and methodically
addresses all potential sites that may harbor a missing gland or glands. A properly
constructed initial operative note that accurately documents remaining histologically identified parathyroid glands and regions explored is of utmost importance and
potential value for the re-operative surgeon. An orderly systematic approach to re-
exploration is necessary in these circumstances to locate the missing gland(s) and
limit morbidity. The order in which regions are approached may vary according to
the surgeon; however, it is important that all potential areas be accessed to increase
the chance of success and avoid a failed re-exploration. The author's preference is
to approach each side explored through the VVA via a lateral to medial orientation.
Regions are then addressed in the following manner: the anterior superior mediastinum is dissected first, with careful attention to the thyrothymic ligament and tracheoesophageal groove region adjacent to the recurrent nerve. Cervical thymectomy,
if not performed at initial surgery, is completed at this time. Dissection then turns to
the retropharyngeal, retroesophageal region where blunt dissection within the prevertebral space will allow for digital exploration superiorly above the cricoid carti-
lage and larynx and inferiorly into the posterior mediastinum. Enlarged glands in
this anatomic plane may often be felt by digital palpation before they are seen using
these maneuvers. Next, the thyroid lobe is mobilized, possibly truncating the superior vascular pedicle to allow rotation of the thyroid gland anteromedially so that the
posterior capsule may be thoroughly examined for a folded, lobulated parathyroid

gland under cover of the capsular fascia. Using this technique, the thyroid lobe is palpated for any nodular densities, which may be suspicious for an intrathyroidal or subcapsular parathyroid gland. The carotid sheath is then opened from the superior mediastinum to the hyoid bone, inspecting and palpating for nodular structures within the sheath. Failing identification on the side explored first, the dissection proceeds contralaterally in the same manner, with orderly inspection of all regions noted above. In the event that a bilateral exploration fails to identify the offending gland, thyroid lobotomy/lobectomy may be performed on the side suspected of harboring the offending gland. It is in this situation where surgeon-performed ultrasound, pre- or intraoperatively, may be of the most benefit to help avoid unnecessary thyroid removal.

In the event that all maneuvers described are unsuccessful in identifying the abnormal missing gland, the procedure is terminated and further measures undertaken to the gland's position by imaging or angioinvasive techniques. Mediastinal dissection is not advisable in the immediate setting, owing to lack of localization and length of time required after a thorough bilateral re-exploration. It should be emphasized that re-exploration should not be undertaken unless there is a reasonable potential for success based on localization studies and/or previous documentation which identifies the putative missing gland.

Intraoperative Assessment of Parathyroid Hormone

Intraoperative assessment of parathyroid hormone (IOPTH) represents a useful adjunct in the performance of parathyroid reoperation, both for single and multiple gland disease entities. The usefulness of biochemically confirming the removal of hyperfunctional parathyroid tissue by applying IOPTH becomes apparent when one considers the previous operative procedure(s) performed by the initial surgeon with respect to what was identified/removed and whether normal glands were identified and histopathologically confirmed. The utilization of IOPTH allows the surgeon to determine the physiologic effect of removal of the putative abnormal gland, indicating removal of all hyperfunctional parathyroid tissue provided the appropriate criteria (>50% decline in PTH) is achieved intraoperatively. Should this decrement not be achieved, further exploration proceeds until IOPTH confirms removal of all hyperfunctional tissue.

Thus, the application of IOPTH in re-exploration potentially limits the extent to which surgical dissection is required in the previously operated neck, thereby limiting the possibility of injury to the recurrent laryngeal nerve and iatrogenic hypoparathyroidism due to manipulation/biopsy of normal glands. Another capability of IOPTH is through intraoperative sampling of blood from the internal jugular veins simultaneously in order to determine a gradient difference in PTH levels, thereby indicating on which neck side a hyperfunctional gland resides (Fig. 5.4). This technique may also be employed to potentially identify an ectopically located undescended inferior parathyroid adenoma, or so-called parathymus, which was not identified at the time of initial exploration (Fig. 5.5). Ultimately, the use of IOPTH in all parathyroid explora-

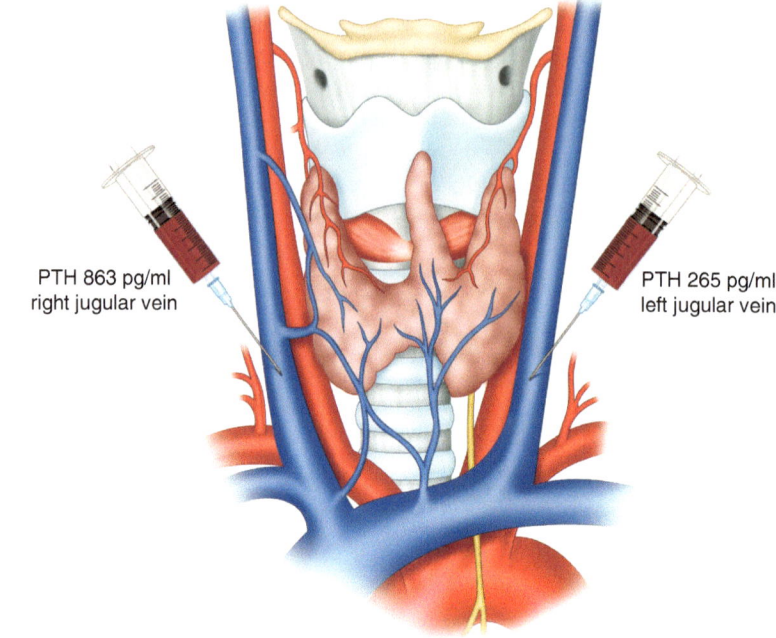

PTH 863 pg/ml
right jugular vein

PTH 265 pg/ml
left jugular vein

Fig. 5.4 Simultaneous IJV sampling for intraoperative PTH assessment

tions provides a measure of biochemical confidence that will serve to limit the extent of surgical dissection and reduce the potential for morbidity.

Mediastinal Exploration

Re-exploration for parathyroid disease may require exploration of the mediastinum. Ectopic parathyroid glands located within the mediastinum and below the level of the thymus account for a small percentage (0.2%) of all abnormally located glands [9]. These inferior parathyroid glands are associated in almost all circumstances with the thymus with which they descend during the embryonic development, having arisen with this structure as a third pharyngeal pouch derivative (Fig. 5.6).

Several approaches to the mediastinum are possible for re-exploration. The choice of approach utilized is dependent on the location of the putative adenoma. Definitive localization is required prior to considering mediastinal surgery. Fusion imaging, combining the anatomic and physiologic capabilities of computed tomography and sestamibi nuclear scintigraphy, provides for simultaneous correlative imaging for hyperfunctional parathyroid glands (Fig. 5.7). The techniques available for approaching the mediastinum include transcervical substernal with cervical

Fig. 5.5 The undescended
inferior parathyroid gland,
so-called parathymus

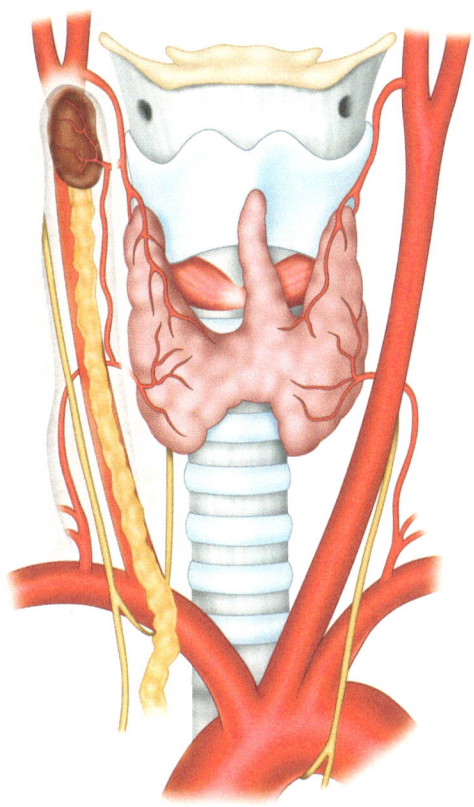

thymectomy using sternal retraction (with or without video assistance) for superior
mediastinal glands, median sternotomy with direct approach to the anterior middle
and caudal compartments, posterolateral thoracotomy for posteriorly based glands
in the lower mediastinal compartment, and video-assisted endoscopic minimally
invasive dissection for selectively focused exploration.

Secondary/Tertiary Hyperparathyroidism and MEN

Recalcitrant hyperparathyroidism following total or subtotal parathyroidectomy in
patients with renal-induced disease represents a unique challenge to the surgeon.
Problems with persistent disease usually result from inadequate resection following
subtotal parathyroidectomy in which three or fewer glands are removed initially or
when supernumerary gland(s) are not recognized during four-gland parathyroidectomy. Recurrent hyperparathyroidism usually results from delayed hyperplasia
developing in cervical parathyroid remnants or within autotransplanted tissue
placed during initial surgery.

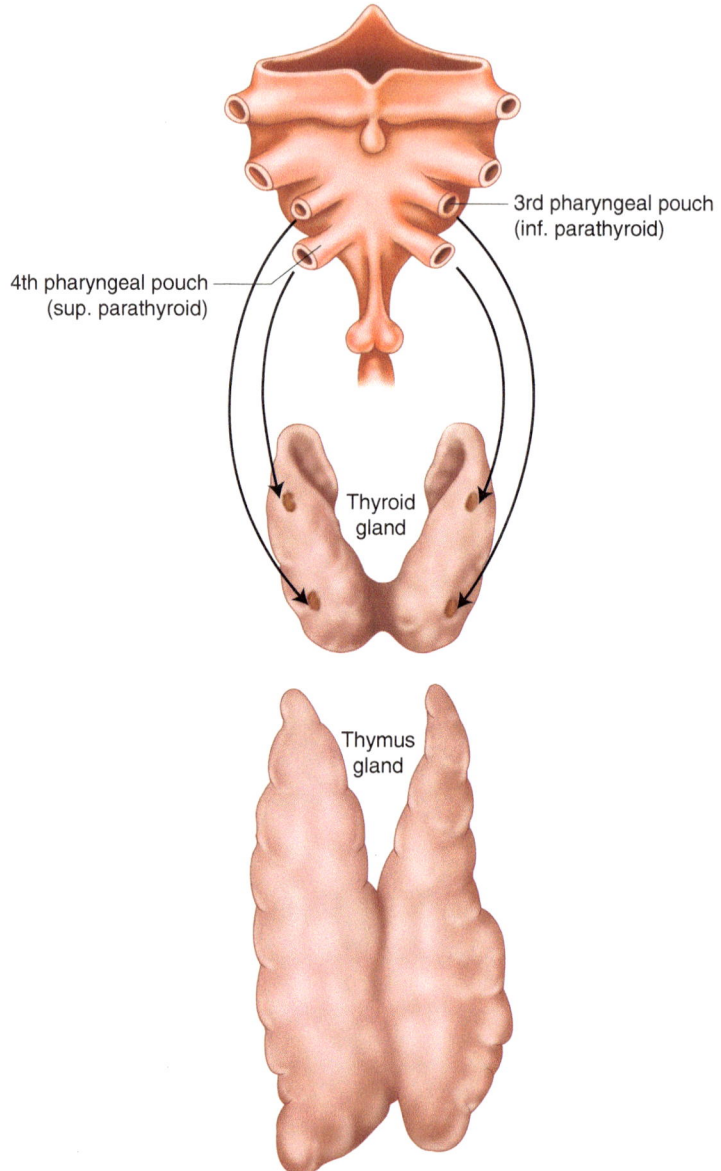

Fig. 5.6 Embryonic derivation of the parathyroid glands

The surgical evaluation for patients recommended for re-exploration includes sestamibi imaging and the determination of the serum PTH gradient in the graft-bearing arm as compared with the contralateral arm in patients who also received autotransplantation initially. Candidate patients in this cohort include those with renal-induced hyperparathyroidism and those with the Multiple endocrine neoplasia type 1 (MEN 1) syndrome in whom total parathyroidectomy was indicated. Patients with the MEN 1 syndrome undergoing re-exploration pose a unique sur-

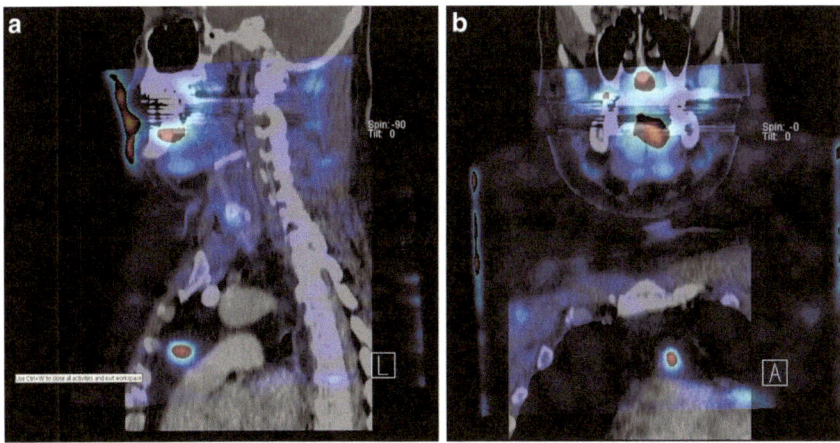

Fig. 5.7 (**a**) Sagittal projection from "fusion" image depicting mediastinal parathyroid adenoma; (**b**) coronal projection of "fusion" image depicting parathyroid adenoma

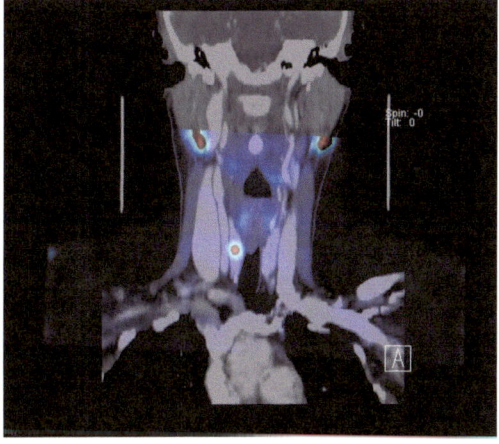

Fig. 5.8 Coronal projection of "fusion" image depicting intrathyroidal parathyroid gland in recurrent MEN 1

Fig. 5.9 Intraoperative photograph depicting the use of the gamma detection device in localizing intrathyroidal parathyroid gland in pt. with recurrent MEN 1

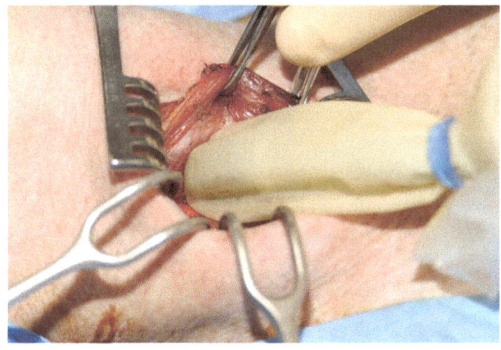

gical challenge in that, even after initial four-gland removal, the possibility of hyperfunctional supernumerary parathyroid tissue exists together with autograft hyperfunction. Unlike sporadic four-gland hyperplasia in patients with primary hyperparathyroidism, those patients with recalcitrant renal- or MEN 1-induced disease will often localize accurately with nuclear scanning (Fig. 5.8). In these instances, the gamma detection device may be utilized to facilitate the dissection in order to limit disturbance to critical surrounding structures and limit morbidity (Fig. 5.9).

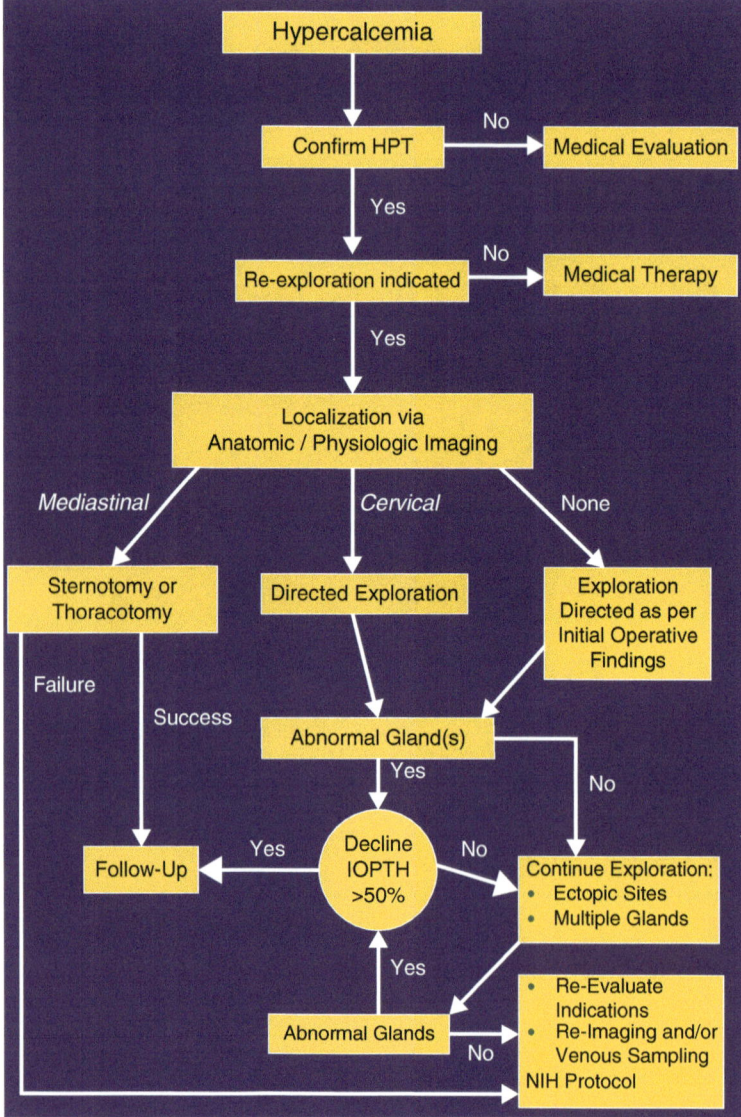

Fig. 5.10 Treatment algorithm for recalcitrant hyperparathyroidism

Summary

Management of recalcitrant hyperparathyroidism represents a unique therapeutic challenge. Opportunity for success and potential morbidity incurred as a result of reoperation differ significantly when compared with initial surgery. The utilization of surgical adjuncts such as invasive/noninvasive localization studies, IOPTH, and gamma probe offers benefit in the management of patients with recurrent hyperparathyroidism. A management protocol is summarized in the treatment algorithm illustrated in Fig. 5.10.

References

1. Haff RC, Ballinger WF. Causes of recurrent hypercalcemia after parathyroidectomy for primary hyperparathyroidism. Ann Surg. 1971;173:884–91.
2. Clark OH, Way LW, Hunt TK. Recurrent hyperparathyroidism. Ann Surg. 1976;184:391–9.
3. Martin JK, van Heerden JA, Edis AJ, et al. Persistent postoperative hyperparathyroidism. Surg Gynecol Obstet. 1980;151:764–8.
4. Jaskowiak N, Norton JA, Alexander HR, Doppman JL, et al. A prospective trail evaluating a standard approach to re-operation for missed parathyroid adenoma. Ann Surg. 1996;224:308–22.
5. ReMine SG. Management of recurrent or persistent hyperparathyroidism. Probl Gen Surg. 1985;2:440–9.
6. Lang JR, Norton JA. Surgery for persistent or recurrent hyperparathyroidism. Curr Pract Surg. 1992;4:56–62.
7. Peeler BB, Martin WH, Sandler MP, et al. Sestamibi parathyroid scanning and postoperative localization studies for patients with recurrent/persistent hyperparathyroidism or significant comorbid conditions: development of an optimal localization strategy. Am Surg. 1997;63:37–46.
8. Tenta LT, Keyes GR. Transcervical parathyroidectomy microsurgical autotransplantation and viscerovertebral arm. Otolaryngol Clin N Am. 1980;13:167–79.
9. Gilmour JR. The gross anatomy of the parathyroid glands. J Pathol. 1938;46:133–49.

Chapter 6
Surgical Techniques and Pearls: The Unsuccessful Reoperation

Jeffrey M. Bumpous and Mary Worthen

Introduction

Even in the most skilled of hands, a small percentage of patients will not be cured after reoperative parathyroid surgery. Reoperative parathyroid surgery can be dangerous even for the most experienced surgeons and is associated with higher complication rates. Damage to the recurrent laryngeal nerve (RLN), hypoparathyroidism, and persistent hyperparathyroidism are the common complications associated with reoperative parathyroid surgery [1]. Reoperative parathyroid surgery is often indicated for persistent primary hyperparathyroidism and recurrent primary hyperparathyroidism. Persistent primary hyperparathyroidism is defined as a failure of serum calcium and parathyroid hormone (PTH) normalization after a parathyroidectomy operation. Recurrent primary hyperparathyroidism occurs when serum calcium and PTH levels are initially normal but become elevated 6 months after surgery [2]. This is common in patients who have undergone a subtotal parathyroidectomy without correction of the underlying abnormality, such as renal disease. This represents a separate entity and will not be considered an unsuccessful operation.

Unsuccessful reoperative parathyroid surgery can result from the misdiagnosis of hyperparathyroidism, the failure to identify affected parathyroid glands radiographically or surgically, incomplete or inappropriate use/interpretation of intraoperative PTH measurements, and lack of adequate postsurgical follow-up. Lack of surgical experience and surgery performed at low-volume surgical centers have shown to have increased rates of unsuccessful repeat surgery [3]. This chapter aims to review common causes of reoperative parathyroid surgery failure with hopes to improve surgical outcomes in this difficult patient population.

J.M. Bumpous (✉) • M. Worthen
Department of Otolaryngology, Head and Neck Surgery and Communicative Disorders,
University of Louisville School of Medicine, Louisville, KY 40202, USA
e-mail: jmbump01@louisville.edu

© Springer International Publishing AG 2018   53
R.P. Tufano, P.K. Pellitteri (eds.), *Reoperative Parathyroid Surgery*,
DOI 10.1007/978-3-319-60723-8_6

Misdiagnosis

Obtaining the correct diagnosis of primary hyperparathyroidism is crucial to successful reoperative parathyroid surgery. Given the increased morbidity associated with re-exploration, the threshold for surgery in remedial operations should be more stringent than for patients undergoing primary surgery. Several diagnoses must be ruled out prior to proceeding with repeat surgery to avoid poor surgical outcomes. Endocrine disorders can mimic primary hyperthyroidism, and a careful preoperative workup is necessary to prevent unsuccessful reoperations or unnecessary operations. In one study, 144 patients who had had previous parathyroid surgery requiring reoperation were evaluated with hopes of improving success rates in parathyroid reoperations. Successful reoperation was defined by prolonged reversal of hypercalcemia. The most common cause of recurrent hyperparathyroidism in their cohort was multiple endocrine neoplasia type 1 (MEN1). Failure of adequate preoperative family history can lead to the failed diagnosis of this disorder, resulting in persistent or recurrent hyperparathyroidism. MEN1 is associated with multiglandular, ectopic, and supernumerary disease. The presence of the syndrome is often not evident at the time of primary operation but can be revealed in prolonged follow-up [4]. The optimal surgical treatment for MEN1 is frequently under debate, but typically involves either total or subtotal parathyroidectomy. Persistent hyperparathyroidism is more frequent after subtotal parathyroidectomy than after total parathyroidectomy with autologous graft of parathyroid tissue. Recurrent hyperparathyroidism has a similar frequency in the two surgical strategies. Genetic testing should be performed on all young patients diagnosed with hyperparathyroidism [5]. In one study, outcomes for 130 consecutive remedial parathyroid explorations were reviewed, resulting in seven failed reoperations due to persistent disease. Four of these patients had multi-gland hyperplasia, one was diagnosed with multiple endocrine neoplasia type 2A (MEN 2A), and one had an occult supernumerary gland after four gland excisions [6].

Not only can unsuccessful parathyroid surgery be secondary to misdiagnosis of primary hyperparathyroidism, certain diseases can mimic normocalcemia in postoperative patients leading to the false belief that the patient has been cured. Similarly, a surgical cure can be incorrectly considered unsuccessful and lead to unnecessary reoperations if not monitored closely. When using surgical adjuncts such as intraoperative PTH (ioPTH) assays as criteria for intraoperative success, it is important to be aware of factors that can falsely alter the measurement. For example, in one large study, younger patients were found to have lower preoperative serum calcium, PTH levels, and ioPTH levels than older patients [7]. Metabolic disorders and poor renal function may falsely elevate the ioPTH. Vitamin D is a known inhibitor of PTH secretion and cause of secondary hyperparathyroidism. These patients may experience deceptive normocalcemia and elevated PTH after parathyroidectomy and have also been shown to have larger adenoma size [8]. These findings may play a role in failure of reoperative parathyroid surgery and support postoperative Vitamin D supplementation in this population [7, 9, 10].

Failure to formulate a well-rounded differential diagnosis and accurately diagnose causes of hypercalcemia and/or hyperparathyroidism can lead to poor outcomes and failure of repeat surgical operations for this population of patients. The differential diagnosis includes hypercalcemia of malignancy, which can falsely elevate calcium and PTH levels. Measurement of an intact PTH (iPTH) level can aid in the differentiation of these diseases; iPTH is generally low in hypercalcemia of malignancy. Familial hypocalciuric hypercalcemia (FHH) is an autosomal dominant disorder that is imperative to diagnose correctly as parathyroidectomy is not indicated for this disorder. An abnormal calcium-sensing receptor characterizes this disease, leading to hypercalcemia, normal or high PTH, and low urinary calcium excretion. The calcium/creatinine clearance is typically <0.01 in FHH [11]. Other important causes of hypercalcemia that the surgeon should be familiar with include exogenous calcium, medications (thiazides and lithium), granulomatous diseases, and metabolic diseases [12].

Failure to Identify Affected Glands Radiographically

Numerous studies have emphasized the need for accurate imaging prior to considering parathyroid surgery. The intraoperative features used to identify parathyroid adenomas such as color, shape, and tactile perception of gland may be much more difficult to appreciate because of fibrosis within the tissues from the previous procedure. For these reasons, most surgeons agree that preoperative imaging studies are an essential component of the workup prior to reoperative parathyroid surgery [13]. Preoperative localization can reduce complication rates and shorten operating time by directing the surgeon to the sites of abnormal glands. The lack of appropriate diagnosis radiographically can lead to unsuccessful reoperative parathyroid surgery.

Recent advances in preoperative localization have led to substantial improved outcomes after remedial surgery. Chen et al. evaluated 254 patients with hyperparathyroidism and found that the positive predictive values for sestamibi scanning, radioguided surgery, and ioPTH testing were 81%, 88%, and 99.5%, respectively [14]. Yen et al. proposed that ultrasonography and sestamibi scans should be performed before all reoperative parathyroid operations [15]. Shen et al. found that the sensitivities of preoperative localization studies were as follows: technetium Tc 99m sestamibi scan, 77%; magnetic resonance imaging, 77%; selective venous catheterization (SVC) for intact parathyroid hormone, 77%; thallium-technetium scan, 68%; ultrasonography (US), 57%; and computed tomography (CT), 42%. The highest false-positive results were found in MRI, and the highest false-negative results were seen in US. Coexisting thyroid disease can often be a confounding variable in both nuclear imaging and high-resolution ultrasound; interpretation of these exams by experienced radiologist and surgeons is of paramount importance. MRI, thallium-technetium, and technetium sestamibi scans were more sensitive for ectopically located tumors than tumors found in normal positions. They concluded that patients who require a reoperation should receive preoperative localization with the combination of noninvasive imaging methods including US, MRI, CT and sestamibi scans; when used together, they correctly identified abnormal glands in 87% of cases. After a failed primary parathyroidectomy, artifacts from surgical clips placed in the neck often limit the diagnostic quality of CT, although it can be useful for evaluation of altered anatomy [16]. Previous studies have demonstrated limited success in locating mediastinal, retrotracheal, retroesophageal, or small adenomas [2]. If radiographic localization remains equivocal after the previous modalities have been performed, then invasive SVC is recommended. This combination of invasive and noninvasive studies identified abnormal glands in 95% of cases [2, 13]. In one large prospective trial performed at the National Institutes of Health (NIH), the results of preoperative imaging protocols and surgical re-exploration in a series of patients with missed parathyroid adenomas after failed initial procedures for primary hyperparathyroidism were evaluated. The highest false-positive results were seen in ultrasonography, likely due to the identification of lymph nodes within the neck. The study concluded that the single best noninvasive imaging study was the sestamibi scan. Sestamibi with 99mTc is the most commonly used radiotracer for imaging of the parathyroid glands. Sestamibi is taken up by both the thyroid and the parathyroid glands, but hyperactive parathyroid tissue retains the radiotracer longer than normal thyroid tissue on delayed images [16]. As a single test, the sestamibi scan has the advantage of relatively low cost, very good sensitivity, and high specificity. Coexisting thyroid disease such as multinodular goiter, autoimmune thyroiditis, and well-differentiated thyroid cancers can be confounding factors decreasing the identification accuracy of technetium sestamibi. Previous studies have described the accuracy of sestamibi scanning in identifying single adenomas to be approximately 99% [17]. Single-photon emission computed tomography (SPECT) can help to differentiate parathyroid activity from overlying thyroid and has been shown to increase sensitivity of scintigraphic parathyroid imaging [16]. The aforementioned study and several others have concluded the optimal combination would be ultrasound (better intrathyroidal evaluation than sestamibi) and sestamibi (improved mediastinal evaluation) [18, 19]. With regard to invasive studies, venous sampling showed a higher rate of true-positive results versus angiography and should be considered when noninvasive studies are inconclusive, as they are expensive and dependent on the skill of the interventional radiologist [13]. Selective venous sampling has been shown to correctly identify the side of affected gland in >89% of cases [20]. Ultrasound-guided parathyroid FNA provides an alternative technique for identification of abnormal glands, in particular intrathyroidal glands. The addition of on-site PTH analysis aids the ultrasonographer by providing real-time feedback and improves accuracy [6]. Although it has been stated that one should not perform remedial parathyroid surgery unless two preoperative imaging studies are both positive and concordant, many accept a positive sestamibi alone as adequate imaging [6]. Interestingly, investigations have shown that surgeon-performed cervical ultrasonography improved the localization of abnormal parathyroid glands preoperatively [21]. Although ultrasound and scintigraphy are established studies for preoperative localization of parathyroid adenomas, four-dimensional computed tomography (4D-CT) has been increasingly adopted and is routinely used at many hospitals [22]. These images provide anatomical and functional information by incorporating perfusion characteristics of hyperfunctioning glands. One recent study compared scintigraphy to 4D-CT in 40 patients and found that the CT correctly localized 76% of parathyroid lesions in 80% of patients and scintigraphy correctly localized 43% of lesions in 48% of patients. Both modalities missed 20% of lesions. Importantly, in patients with prior failed parathyroidectomies, 4D-CT correctly identified lesions in all five patients, and scintigraphy missed two lesions. The smallest lesion detected by 4D-CT was 4 mm and 10 mm for scintigraphy. 4D-CT exposes the patient to significantly higher doses of ionizing radiation [23]. Four phases may not be necessary; Noureldine et al. found that two-phase and four-phase CT provide an equivalent diagnostic accuracy in localizing hyperfunctional parathyroid glands. The reduced radiation exposure to the patient may make two-phase acquisitions a more acceptable alternative for preoperative localization [24]. To improve unsuccessful reoperative parathyroid surgery, continued research in the radiographic diagnosis of parathyroid lesions is warranted.

Intraoperative Failure to Identify Affected Glands

Aberrant parathyroid tissues are more likely to deviate from the typical anatomic positions of normal parathyroid tissue in patients who have previously had neck surgery. An unsuccessful reoperation may be secondary to ectopic parathyroid tissue, hyperplasia, supernumerary glands, or inadequate/partially resected normal parathyroid adenoma which can result in parathyromatosis. An ectopic parathyroid gland may be hidden anywhere from the pericardium up to the nasal septum. A normal superior gland position is defined as the region posterolateral to the superior pole of the thyroid superior and posterior to the course of the RLN. The normal inferior gland position is defined as in the region of the lower pole of the thyroid gland anterior to the RLN and the inferior thyroid artery [13]. Shen et al. evaluated 102 failed parathyroid operations and found that ectopic parathyroid tissue was present in >50% of reoperative cases. Thirty-seven percent of cases resulted from the incomplete resection of multi-gland disease, and 7% were due to the lack of identification of an adenoma in a normal location. Similar to previous studies, the majority of ectopic glands were found in the paraesophageal region (28%), non-thymic mediastinal region, (26%), intrathymic region (24%), and intrathyroidal region (11%), within the carotid sheath (9%), and in high cervical position (2%). Five patients had unsuccessful reoperations, and two of these had multiple supernumerary glands in ectopic positions in the mediastinum. All five had false-positive localization studies [2]. Lesions in the tracheoesophageal groove/posterior superior mediastinum can be considered to be in the normal position of the superior parathyroid gland; therefore, it is not considered a true ectopic site. It is not uncommon for adenomas to be adherent to the undersurface of the RLN in this region. Reluctance to dissect near the nerve can be a major factor in the failure to appreciate superior parathyroid glands in this region. In one prospective study, 222 consecutive patients who underwent re-exploration for hyperparathyroidism at the National Institutes of Health (NIH) were evaluated. The most common site for a missed adenoma was in the tracheoesophageal groove in the posterior superior mediastinum, and the most common ectopic site was the thymus or mediastinum. 13 of the 222 initial reoperations failed the procedure, with six patients requiring another procedure. One patient had diffuse muscular seeding in the strap and sternocleidomastoid muscles (parathyromatosis). Successful extirpation of diseased parathyroid tissue in these cases may require expansion of the resection to include non-parathyroidal adjacent tissues in order to reestablish calcium homeostasis; the trade-off however is that operative morbidity may be increased. The other five patients were re-explored 6 months after the initial procedure. Repeat imaging workup in three patients showed unusual abnormal gland locations in the nasopharynx and aortopulmonary window. Two failed the procedure when intrathyroidal tissue was incorrectly identified as being adenomas on frozen section. Seventeen patients with failed reoperations developed recurrent disease at much later dates (>6 months). Most parathyroid glands were found to regrow at the site of initial surgical resection, and seven had recurrent disease in a single lesion on the contralateral side of earlier abnormal lesion; this entity has been described to be a double adenoma [13]. It must be emphasized that a surgeon who performs a unilateral exploration runs the risk of missing a second adenoma or hyperplastic glands even if ioPTH is used. MEN1 has increased frequency of supernumerary glands and ectopic glands, and embryonic rests can be embedded within fatty tissue surrounding the trachea, esophagus, and carotid artery [5]. Patients with MEN1 frequently present at age less than 40 years as well; so the threshold for consideration of MEN1 should be higher in the younger patient cohort. There is a subset of patients in whom parathyroid glands are not identified during reoperative surgery, potentially leading to an unsuccessful reoperation. In this setting, it is recommended that bilateral explorations be performed to search potential ectopic sites. In addition, if one ectopic parathyroid gland is initially visualized, other possible ectopic sites should be evaluated prior to any removal of parathyroid tissue, such that the existence of single versus multiglandular disease can be more appropriately defined. These sites include the thymus, superior mediastinum, retroesophageal and submandibular regions, carotid sheath, upper cervical region for missing lower gland, and posterior mediastinum for missing upper gland. If all areas are negative, intraoperative ultrasound and bilateral internal jugular vein sampling to determine if an ipsilateral PTH gradient is present should be considered, although ultrasound can be difficult once surgery has started and surgical planes are disrupted. A thyroid lobectomy is an option, with median sternotomy/mediastinoscopy or other thoracic endoscopies reserved for failure to identify the abnormality in all other locations; this could occur coincident to cervical exploration or at a later date considering the overall condition of the patient. If all else fails, ligation of the blood supply to the missing parathyroid gland has been reported, but represents a strategy with limited evidence basis for long-term efficacy [6]. Gamma probe detection of radiolabeled sestamibi has been used to guide cervical dissection in remedial cases. One study experienced successful minimally invasive radioguided parathyroidectomy (MIRP) in reoperative parathyroid surgery using the gamma probe for single adenomas as predicted by sestamibi scan. Current thinking is that minimally invasive surgery when indicated is likely to decrease the risk of nerve injury due to directed technique and less exploration of unnecessary areas while minimizing dissection and can offer a patient avoidance of general anesthesia and perhaps a lower rate of permanent hypoparathyroidism [6, 17].

Pitfalls of the Utilization of the Intraoperative Parathyroid Hormone Assay

Intraoperative parathyroid hormone (ioPTH) assay has allowed surgeons to perform minimally invasive parathyroid surgery with success rates comparable to bilateral exploration and can confirm the removal of all hyperfunctioning parathyroid tissue in a relatively short time period, as the half-life of PTH is approximately 5 min [25]. The earliest method for monitoring ioPTH was described in the 1990s by Irvin et al. [26], who recommended a 50% decline from pre-excision PTH levels at 10 min after gland excision. The commonly applied Irvin criterion is reported to correctly predict postoperative calcium levels in 96–98% of patients. However, when these criteria are met intraoperatively yet persistent hyperparathyroidism occurs, one must question the clinical accuracy of the 50% drop criteria in PTH levels. Other investigators have shown presence of multiglandular disease despite a 50% drop in the ioPTH level. However, the PTH baseline reference concentration can be markedly increased by surgical manipulations during preparation of the affected glands, individual variability of the PTH half-life, and modifications in the physiological state of the patient during surgery such as renal failure [27]. Thus, one could misinterpret an apparent 50% decrement as representing an adequate fall in ioPTH and thereby miss occult residual multi-gland disease [13]. One study evaluated 1882 patients and found that a 10 min post-excision ioPTH level that decreased 50% from baseline and is normal or near normal was highly successful, versus relying on 50% decrease alone. 22.4% of patients with multiglandular disease experienced failed operation when using the 50% decrease alone [28]. In the challenging reoperative patient, unsuccessful reoperation may be attributed to failure of accurately evaluating the ioPTH degradation curve. Accordingly, more stringent criteria have been appropriately described for an intraoperative definition of cure in the reoperative scenario. A measurement of a 10 and 20 min value could contribute to the identification of patients eligible for avoidance of further neck exploration in a previously operated neck with higher risk of surgical complications [29]. When used for the discrimination of hyperparathyroidism caused by hyperplasia or multiglandular disease such as in MEN1, ioPTH has shown substantially lower reliability, with a high rate of false-positive values [5]. One retrospective review evaluated 1371 patients undergoing ioPTH monitoring and found that persistent and recurrent disease rate was lowest in the patient with final ioPTH <40 pg/mL [7]. Another study evaluated

1108 individuals with a mean follow-up of 1.8 years and found that patients with final ioPTH levels <40 pg/mL also had lower recurrence rates [30]. Baseline index PTH levels can alert the surgeon to the potential for the presence of multi-gland disease. Baseline levels below 100 pg/ml in patients with hyperparathyroidism often indicate, low volume, single gland disease [31]. The failure to obtain final ioPTH level < 40 pg/mL by surgeons may partially be responsible for an unsuccessful operation, especially in the absence of bilateral exploration. Of all the perioperative adjuncts used during parathyroid surgery, intraoperative PTH testing has the highest sensitivity, positive predictive value, and accuracy. Although important for preoperative evaluation, imaging modalities allow the surgeon to localize the abnormality, but ioPTH evaluation are crucial in assessing results of surgery and emphasize the critical importance of close follow-up after surgery [14].

Incomplete Follow-Up

Postoperative reoperative parathyroid surgical patients must be carefully monitored for surgical complications. Intraoperative PTH values not only provide valuable intraoperative information for the surgeon but can also be used as a guide for follow-up plan. ioPTH levels greater than 40 have been shown to experience higher rates of persistence and recurrence, and recurrence may not be evident until roughly 2 years after surgery or longer. It is therefore imperative to perform close surveillance for patients who meet this criteria to avoid unsuccessful reoperations [7].

Reoperative patients are at higher risk for inadequate postoperative parathyroid function and RLN paralysis. Postoperative hypocalcemia is often temporary; most patients becoming hypocalcemic will improve, while normal residual parathyroid tissue regains function in the first several days after reoperation. A subset of patients, however, will remain hypocalcemic and will require lifelong calcium and vitamin D replacement. A possible cause of unsuccessful reoperative parathyroid surgery defined by postoperative complications is due to incomplete initial workup and/or follow-up. Laryngoscopic evaluation of bilateral RLN function is a critical component of the preoperative evaluation, even if the patient is asymptomatic. The knowledge of a RLN injury is likely to impact the choice of operative approach in the remedial setting. Close monitoring of calcium and PTH levels is critical in a reoperative patient. Long-term follow-up must be especially performed in patients with endocrine disorders (MEN) as they are at higher risk for recurrent hyperparathyroidism [4]. If persistent or recurrent disease is biochemically confirmed, the patient must be carefully reassessed as a new patient. This includes repeat history and physical examination, repeat laryngoscopic evaluation, preoperative imaging (often multimodal), and laboratory values including 24 h urine calcium. Given that the risk of surgical complication increases with each repeat exploration, truly asymptomatic reoperative patients with unsuccessful surgery with borderline laboratory abnormalities may be considered for nonoperative management [25].

References

1. Richards ML, Thompson GB, Farley DR, Grant CS. Reoperative parathyroidectomy in 228 patients during the era of minimal-access surgery and intraoperative parathyroid hormone monitoring. Am J Surg. 2008;196:937–42. discussion 942–933
2. Shen W, Duren M, Morita E, et al. Reoperation for persistent or recurrent primary hyperparathyroidism. Arch Surg. 1996;131:861–7. discussion 867–869
3. Chen H, Wang TS, Yen TW, et al. Operative failures after parathyroidectomy for hyperparathyroidism: the influence of surgical volume. Ann Surg. 2010;252:691–5.
4. Hessman O, Stalberg P, Sundin A, et al. High success rate of parathyroid reoperation may be achieved with improved localization diagnosis. World J Surg. 2008;32:774–81. discussion 782–773
5. Tonelli F, Giudici F, Cavalli T, Brandi ML. Surgical approach in patients with hyperparathyroidism in multiple endocrine neoplasia type 1: total versus partial parathyroidectomy. Clinics (Sao Paulo). 2012;67(Suppl 1):155–60.
6. Udelsman R, Donovan PI. Remedial parathyroid surgery: changing trends in 130 consecutive cases. Ann Surg. 2006;244:471–9.
7. Rajaei MH, Bentz AM, Schneider DF, Sippel RS, Chen H, Oltmann SC. Justified follow-up: a final intraoperative parathyroid hormone (ioPTH) over 40 pg/mL is associated with an increased risk of persistence and recurrence in primary hyperparathyroidism. Ann Surg Oncol. 2015;22:454–9.
8. Beyer TD, Solorzano CC, Prinz RA, Babu A, Nilubol N, Patel S. Oral vitamin D supplementation reduces the incidence of eucalcemic PTH elevation after surgery for primary hyperparathyroidism. Surgery. 2007;141:777–83.
9. Carsello CB, Yen TW, Wang TS. Persistent elevation in serum parathyroid hormone levels in normocalcemic patients after parathyroidectomy: does it matter? Surgery. 2012;152:575–81. discussion 581-573
10. Untch BR, Barfield ME, Dar M, Dixit D, Leight GS Jr, Olson JA Jr. Impact of 25-hydroxyvitamin D deficiency on perioperative parathyroid hormone kinetics and results in patients with primary hyperparathyroidism. Surgery. 2007;142:1022–6.
11. Fuleihan Gel H. Familial benign hypocalciuric hypercalcemia. J Bone Miner Res. 2002;17(Suppl 2):N51–6.
12. Fuleihan G, Silverberg SJ. In: Rosen C, editor. Primary hyperparathyroidism: diagnosis, differential diagnosis, and evaluation. Waltham, MA: UpToDate; 2016. Accessed 25 Jun 2016.
13. Jaskowiak N, Norton JA, Alexander HR, et al. A prospective trial evaluating a standard approach to reoperation for missed parathyroid adenoma. Ann Surg. 1996;224:308–20. discussion 320–301
14. Chen H, Mack E, Starling JR. A comprehensive evaluation of perioperative adjuncts during minimally invasive parathyroidectomy: which is most reliable? Ann Surg. 2005;242:375–80. discussion 380–373
15. Yen TW, Wang TS, Doffek KM, Krzywda EA, Wilson SD. Reoperative parathyroidectomy: an algorithm for imaging and monitoring of intraoperative parathyroid hormone levels that results in a successful focused approach. Surgery. 2008;144:611–9. discussion 619–621
16. Johnson NA, Tublin ME, Ogilvie JB. Parathyroid imaging: technique and role in the preoperative evaluation of primary hyperparathyroidism. AJR Am J Roentgenol. 2007;188:1706–15.
17. Norman J, Denham D. Minimally invasive radioguided parathyroidectomy in the reoperative neck. Surgery. 1998;124:1088–92. discussion 1092-1083
18. Solorzano CC, Carneiro-Pla DM, Irvin GL III. Surgeon-performed ultrasonography as the initial and only localizing study in sporadic primary hyperparathyroidism. J Am Coll Surg. 2006;202:18–24.
19. Lumachi F, Zucchetta P, Marzola MC, et al. Advantages of combined technetium-99m-sestamibi scintigraphy and high-resolution ultrasonography in parathyroid localization:

comparative study in 91 patients with primary hyperparathyroidism. Eur J Endocrinol. 2000;143:755–60.
20. Lebastchi AH, Aruny JE, Donovan PI, et al. Real-time super selective venous sampling in remedial parathyroid surgery. J Am Coll Surg. 2015;220:994–1000.
21. Solorzano CC, Lee TM, Ramirez MC, Carneiro DM, Irvin GL. Surgeon-performed ultrasound improves localization of abnormal parathyroid glands. Am Surg. 2005;71:557–62. discussion 562–553
22. Hoang JK, Williams K, Gaillard F, Dixon A, Sosa JA. Parathyroid 4D-CT: multi-institutional international survey of use and trends. Otolaryngol Head Neck Surg. 2016;155(6):956–60.
23. Galvin L, Oldan JD, Bahl M, Eastwood JD, Sosa JA, Hoang JK. Parathyroid 4D CT and scintigraphy: what factors contribute to missed parathyroid lesions? Otolaryngol Head Neck Surg. 2016;154:847–53.
24. Noureldine SI, Aygun N, Walden MJ, Hassoon A, Gujar SK, Tufano RP. Multiphase computed tomography for localization of parathyroid disease in patients with primary hyperparathyroidism: how many phases do we really need? Surgery. 2014;156:1300–6. discussion 13006–13007
25. Prescott JD, Udelsman R. Remedial operation for primary hyperparathyroidism. World J Surg. 2009;33:2324–34.
26. Irvin GL III, Dembrow VD, Prudhomme DL. Operative monitoring of parathyroid gland hyperfunction. Am J Surg. 1991;162:299–302.
27. Calo PG, Pisano G, Loi G, et al. Intraoperative parathyroid hormone assay during focused parathyroidectomy: the importance of 20 minutes measurement. BMC Surg. 2013;13:36.
28. Richards ML, Thompson GB, Farley DR, Grant CS. An optimal algorithm for intraoperative parathyroid hormone monitoring. Arch Surg. 2011;146:280–5.
29. Di Stasio E, Carrozza C, Pio Lombardi C, et al. Parathyroidectomy monitored by intraoperative PTH: the relevance of the 20 min end-point. Clin Biochem. 2007;40:595–603.
30. Wharry LI, Yip L, Armstrong MJ, et al. The final intraoperative parathyroid hormone level: how low should it go? World J Surg. 2014;38:558–63.
31. Clark MJ, Pellitteri PK. Assessing the impact of low baseline parathyroid hormone levels on surgical treatment of primary hyperparathyroidism. Laryngoscope. 2009;119:1100–5.

Index

© Springer International Publishing AG 2018

63

R.P. Tufano, P.K. Pellitteri (eds.), *Reoperative Parathyroid Surgery*,
DOI 10.1007/978-3-319-60723-8